A Daily Walk

A Daily Walk in the Temple

90 Day Wellness Guide & Journal

SPIRIT, MIND, AND BODY

Maddie Frazier

Xulon Press Elite
555 Winderley Pl, Suite 225
Maitland, FL 32751
407.339.4217
www.xulonpress.com

Xulon Elite

© 2024 by Maddie Frazier

All rights reserved solely by the author. The author guarantees all contents are original and do not infringe upon the legal rights of any other person or work. No part of this book may be reproduced in any form without the permission of the author.

Due to the changing nature of the Internet, if there are any web addresses, links, or URLs included in this manuscript, these may have been altered and may no longer be accessible. The views and opinions shared in this book belong solely to the author and do not necessarily reflect those of the publisher. The publisher therefore disclaims responsibility for the views or opinions expressed within the work.

Unless otherwise indicated, Scripture quotations taken from the Holy Bible, New International Version (NIV). Copyright © 1973, 1978, 1984, 2011 by Biblica, Inc.™. Used by permission. All rights reserved.

Paperback ISBN-13: 978-1-66289-300-1
eBook ISBN-13: 978-1-66289-301-8

Preface

IF YOU HAVE recently purchased this Spiritual and Wellness Journal, I congratulate you on your new journey. Two years ago in 2021, I was walking on a beach in South Carolina halfway through a wellness challenge. This challenge brought me closer to God which was something I truly was not expecting. I am not sure that the creator of this challenge had a spiritual change in mind. As I was walking down the beach God was speaking to me about the talents and gifts, He had imparted in me. One was my passion to help people improve their quality of life through wellness coaching. The other was my ability to edify others while lifting them during difficult times. During this walk, God told me I was going to write a book. I remember this day so vividly. I can recall laughing so hard I was crying during this prayer time. Why? Because I am dyslexic. I cannot write a sentence much less a book. I told God for the first time in my life He was crazy. I returned home from this beach trip and said, "ok God, let's do this!" I thought why not take on a challenge and began to research how to write a book. The attempt overwhelmed me, and I gave up. September, the following year, I decided to do the wellness challenge again. It was September of 2022. I was about ten days into this second challenge and God again said I was going to write a book. This time He made sure I knew He was serious! He stuck a person who is an editor in my face! This person has become very precious to me as an editor and even more so a friend. She inspired me to sit down and stop worrying about how it would sound. She told me to pour my heart and spirit out, say what needed to be said, and just write! I can hear her now, "don't worry about the logistics of getting it published start at the beginning." Over the next weeks and months as I was working out, God was pouring into my spirit what to write. It wasn't long before He was sending people to me from all directions who would inspire me and keep me moving forward. I cannot remember a day in my life I did not say anything about wellness. I have felt that God wanted me to help others since I was in the sixth grade. He has been with me all my life. Now God wants me to speak and write. Through this process I found myself relating a lot to Moses. Moses was afraid and stuttered as was I. God gave Moses Aaron to help on his journey the same way he put so many people in my life for this purpose. Knowing the issues I have with speaking and writing, I can definitely attest to the fact that God doesn't always call on the qualified, but He will qualify the called.

I hold certifications in personal training and functional nutrition counseling. This book aims to inspire and guide readers towards realizing their full potential. It emphasizes the importance of prioritizing God in one's journey towards wellness. He created you and lives in you if you have accepted Him as your Lord and Savior. Although I have trained several individuals by utilizing the information and techniques in this book, it is important to note that I am not a licensed medical practitioner. My favorite clients are those that say I cannot change my life. I will always be a couch potato. Well, if you have a desire, and you want to spread the word of God, you have found the right book. I highly recommend you schedule an appointment with your personal physician for a thorough physical before starting this journey. Know your limits before beginning any wellness journey. It is also a good idea to get your bloodwork completed and continue to do so periodically throughout your journey. It is one of the best ways to track your success and see the health benefits you and God are creating. Let your doctor know what your intentions are. Most of us do not want to compete in a show or be a fitness model although it is great if those are your goals. We just want to focus on changing our health and allowing God to move in us, through us, and with us. I look forward to hearing from those that God has inspired and are moving in His light.

Do you know that you are the **TEMPLE** **of GOD** and that the *Spirit of God* dwells in you?.

1 Corinthians 3:16

A Daily Walk in the Temple

Introduction

IT WAS FALL of 1970. Bob and Lynne Sizemore conceived their first child. Bobby was born June 23, 1971. Why is this important? Women have children every day. Well, they were told Lynne would not be able to conceive children, so as a precaution, Lynne decided to get a form of birth control that would stop her from being able to conceive again. However, there is no stopping God! The next Fall, 1972, another baby was conceived. Little did they know what was about to hit their otherwise peaceful life. June 21, 1973, Madeline Christina Sizemore was born.

Yes, me! I was born stubborn and strong-willed from day one. Even as a newborn, I was extremely vocal. I refused to keep my clothes on, and no matter what... I mean no matter what, I wanted my way! I grew into a tomboy that loved to be outside, my happiest memories were when I could play the hardest.

A positive part of my life from as early as I can remember was church. Both my parents and grandparents made sure my brother and I were in church. Sunday mornings, weather permitting, my grandparents, brother, and I would walk to church. These mornings were exciting for me. Each season would bring about new conversations. We would talk about how God created the plants, flowers, and animals we would see. Walking home from church we discussed what we learned in Sunday school. The one-on-one time with my grandparents during these walks was peaceful and full of love.

We attended a Southern Baptist church. Sometimes sermons would really scare me. I remember sitting beside my grandmother many Sunday mornings tucking my head in her arm during sermons talking about hell, fire, brimstone, and satan. I do not know why my brother and I did not attend a children's church. If there were such a thing, we were not in it. I had a keen sense of who God the Father, God the Son, and God the Holy Spirit was at an early age, even though the sermons would scare me at times. I knew the preacher loved me, and he was preaching truth. Wednesdays were the best! We had a children's choir, and singing was my favorite. I am not sure if I sang very well, but I loved to sing. Singing would always bring peace over me.

I can remember one special Sunday morning. The sermon was not so scary, and the Preacher was talking about a prayer closet. He said that Jesus told us to go to our prayer closet when we pray. Basically, do not be lavish and boastful when praying, and humble yourself when you pray. I am sure you could imagine a 4-year old's mind translating this. So, I went home and turned my closet into a place I thought a prayer closet should be. Imagine this cozy scene: I have my cherished blanket and pillows, along with my favorite stuffed animals, all arranged around me. And to complete the picture, I have a small Bible that was given to me for being in a wedding. When I was scared or my mom was upset with me (which was often), I would go to my closet and pray. So, at an early age I knew there was a God, He loved me, and He was in that closet! We met and talked there a lot!

Then life began. Different traumas started to mold who I was. One particular summer, I was around 8 years old, and my brother and I were at the church's daycare. I had a terrible experience that caused me to have a huge fear of being in the church. I was told to get over it and move on. That is exactly what I did. I learned to face my fears incredibly young. But anytime I was alone in the church I would well up in fear. The one place we should feel safe, and when alone I did not.

Around the same time, my brother and I who were previously attending public school, were then placed in a private Christian school. Imagine a tomboy with dyslexia, who despised wearing dresses and skirts, but was made to wear them every day. Little girls made jokes about me. Why don't you brush your hair? Your shoes are dirty, you need to clean them! Why do you speak backwards? You play too rough! The list goes on and on. I learned at an early age to hide my fears. Get big, bold, and loud.

I worked hard to get over how the kids treated me because switching schools was not an option. At this school, I was taught how to speak in public and how to memorize long poems, songs, and bible verses. I was not the best at public speaking. If you are around me long enough, you will hear how I speak backwards and create new words by putting two or three together. To my advantage, I was gaining skills I could use throughout my life. All while God, laid a foundation in my soul and spirit.

This time in my life is when the Trinity became alive to me. Some people run away from God because of kids and people hurting them, or preachers scaring them. I did the opposite. I wanted to be closer. I really started to learn the Word of God. We had to memorize 10 verses a month. 1 Corinthians 13:11 starts; As a child I spoke like a child. I did not fully understand what these verses meant at the time, but God knew what I could comprehend at that age. While building this foundation, we learned about the Temple. I was intrigued by how intricate the Temple was. The courtyard, each room, veil, alter, sacrifices, oils, down to the rope the priest had to wear around his waist were all significant pieces that made up the house of God.

We learned Jesus died on the cross, rose from the dead, and ascended into heaven! The Holy Spirit lives in us! We are now the Temple of God! Well, that blew me away! At the same time this also worried me. I must be perfect! God does not want to live in a dirty house! What if I sinned and dropped dead like the priest did if he was not atoned for his sins and tried to go before God. I tried to be good, but somehow developed a temper instead. I was always in trouble, never was good enough, always talked over by others, and never fit in. Fortunately for me, God was always there. I look back and He would be in that closet. Wiping away my tears and listening to my fears. Forgiving me when I would go into detail asking for forgiveness. Hearing how I felt, He would try so hard to comfort me and help me find positives. Most days it worked as His grace and love overcame all that was bad in the moment.

The summer before starting the seventh grade we left that church and began attending a different church. Not only did we start a new church, my brother and I were placed back into public school. I was so excited! I could stop wearing dresses and was very excited about being reunited with old friends. Well, that was not the case. I had grown spiritually more than I realized. I carried my Bible to each class like I had become accustomed to and quickly found out you did not do that in public school. This Book made me feel safe; however, the kids thought I was strange. I did not stop bringing it to school, but I did leave it in my locker. So, for the first time in my little life, I was hiding Jesus. I began to feel guilty. The church we just started had an awesome youth director who taught me God meets us where we are, and He lives in us. I picked up where I left off and remembered I am the Temple. The word was in me. I had a foundation to stand on.

The reason I started this book with the background of the beginning of my life is because we all carry baggage. We all have trauma. We all have sinned and fallen short of the Glory of God. The coolest thing is He is there holding out His hand ready for us. God is waiting for us to love Him back.

This is where I want to begin helping you with this Journey. Let us go back to being a child.

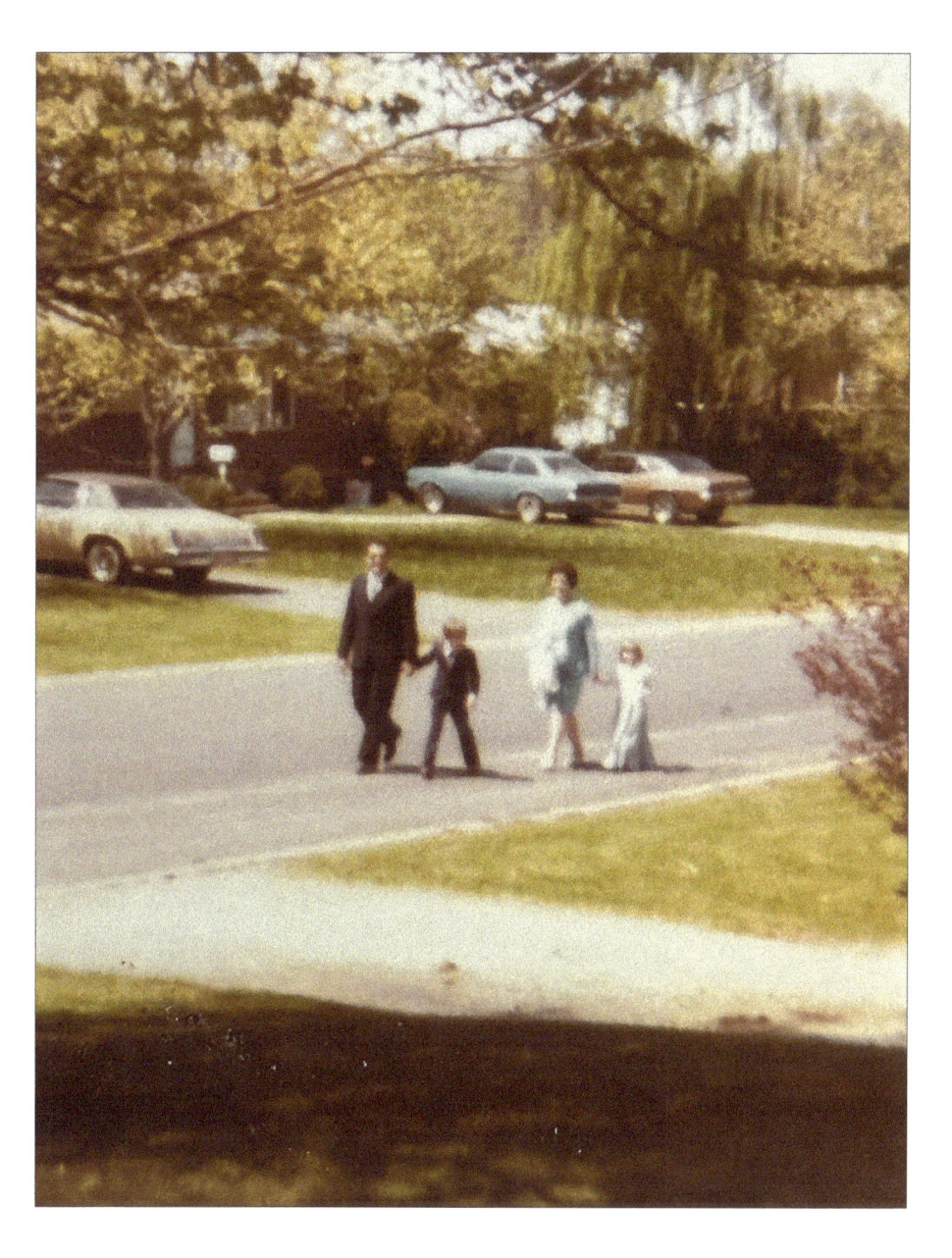

**A Day weather permitted us to walk
to church. Easter morning**

SPIRIT BODY & MIND

90 day wellness journal

LE'S GET STARTED

Let us clean our Temples.
Spirit, Mind and Body.

What can you expect over the next 90 days?

FIRST AND MOST importantly, I pray you will experience a change in your relationship with God. You will begin to hear His voice and feel His presence. When you wake in the morning, you will be filled with a desire to be in the Word and prayer before anything else, and you will make it happen.

Second, your thought process should begin to be more positive. You will learn to hold your thoughts captive and take them in a positive direction. You will start seeing value in your thoughts, in the people around you, and your activities throughout the day.

The third expectation is twofold. Becoming accustomed to eating cleaner and making healthier choices will become easier by the end of the 90 days. WE STRIVE FOR PROGRESS NOT PERFECTION! The second part of this is you should begin to see physical changes. Visible changes will vary depending on where you were physically from day one. Some will see they can walk more and be less out of breath. Some will see clothes fitting better. Some may even need to purchase a new wardrobe.

Remember, each person is on his or her own journey. We cannot look to our right or our left and try to be those people. We need to seek God and find what He created us to be.

Spirit
& MIND

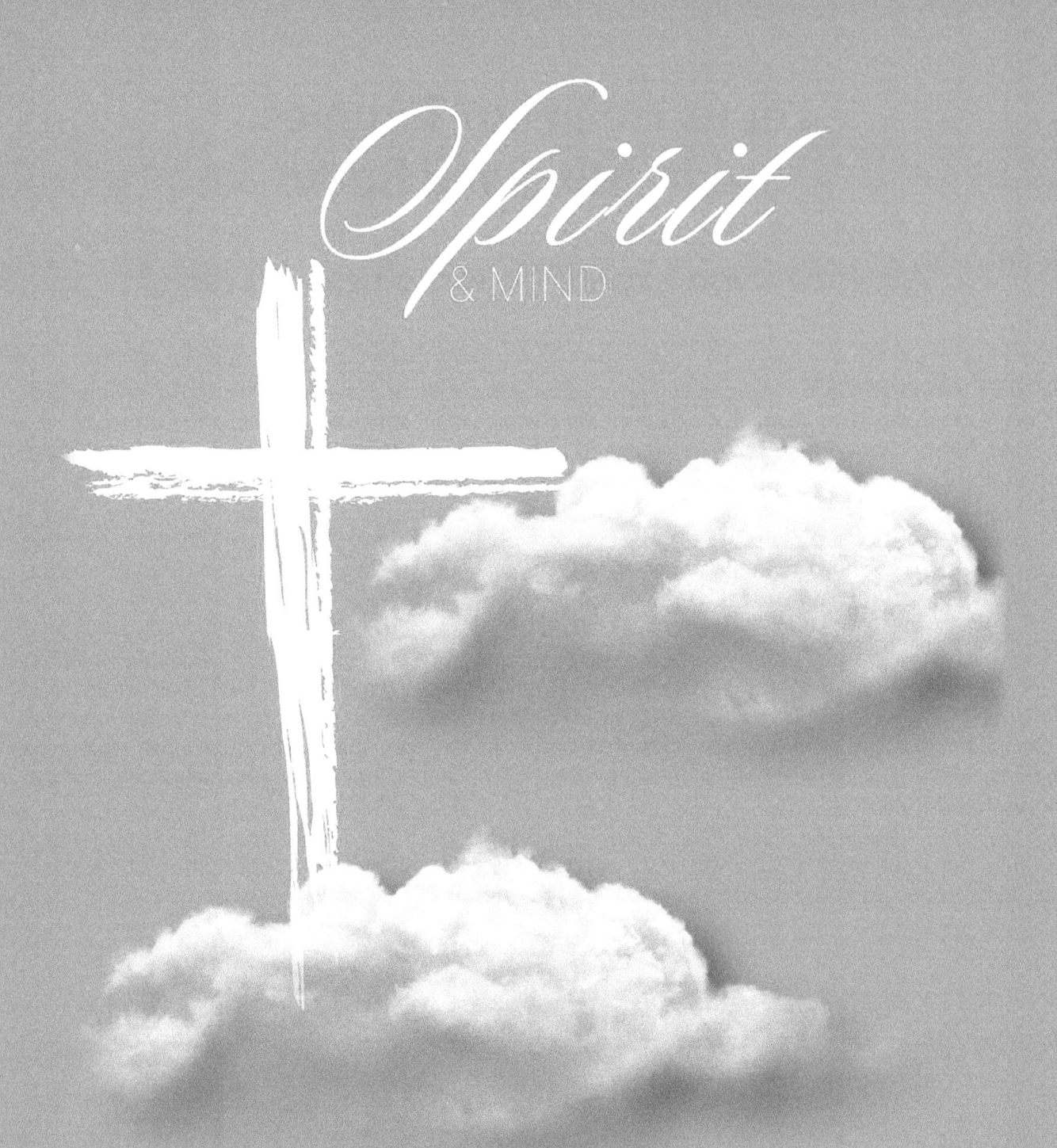

Ephesians 4:23 Be renewed in the spirit of your mind, and that you put on the new man which was created according to God, in true righteousness, holiness.

Spirit and Mind

GOD'S SPIRIT DWELLS within us. Wow! That is amazing. Have you ever sat down and really thought about what that means? First, the Spirit walks with you, eats with you, moves with you, and sleeps with you. Second, the POWER is within you! I think of the pop song from 2003 by SNAP that's titled, I'VE GOT THE POWER! This is you all day and every day! YOU'VE GOT THE POWER! Therefore, if the Spirit is in you and the POWER is in you, why are you not taping into this? Why are you not keeping the Spirits home as perfect as you can?

Well, Tina, how do I do this? You will not believe this! It is so simple! The answer is to pray! That is the first thing you do. Secondly, read and meditate on the Word of God daily. I believe spending fifteen to twenty minutes a day in the Word is worth every second. He does not ask a lot. He just wants to talk to you. Using this devotional, you will take fifteen to twenty minutes each morning with God. Read a part of the word and reflect on it. Journal your thoughts, prayer request, and how you feel. Tell God each day three things you are grateful for. Tell God these things each morning. Plug into the power that dwells in you. When you least expect it, you will begin to hear His voice. You will begin to feel His power stirring within you.

Taking this time each morning with God will begin to change your mind. The way you think will become more positive. Positive thoughts bring positive actions. Our mind is a powerful part of our life. We move throughout the day because our mind leads us in a direction. Our mind dictates what we say, what we do, and where we go. If we constantly have a negative outlook, we will always have a negative day. Spending time in God's Word each morning, will start you off with a positive mindset. If we are thinking positively, we do not have room for negativity. Therefore, we speak and move in positive ways.

Remember

YOU'VE GOT THE POWER!

BODY
FOOD & MOVEMENT
A Daily Commitment

Body: Food and Movement

FOOD

NOW THAT WE have covered the Sprit and mind, we need to know how to treat the temple. Our temple is the one and only body God gave us while we are here on earth. We live in a world with so many toxic chemicals that are "Food and Drug Administration (FDA) approved". There are products that say "natural" or "low fat". We have been trained to think these are good for us. In the 1950s, we started eating processed foods. Imitation foods that are full of preservatives. Then, by the 1980s, we went into a "fat free" generation, switching fat with sugar and carbohydrates. Now, in the 2000s, we have countless numbers of trendy diets. These diets range from keto, Atkins, low carb, high protein, vegan, vegetarian, and carnivore. The list goes on and on ad nauseum. While some of the trends have merit, none of them will give us what we are really looking for, which is "a quick fix."

What we really need to do is go back to the basics: fruits, vegetables, and clean meats. What did we eat before grocery stores? Did we eat twinkies and fast food? We ate fresh foods, fruits and vegetables that were in season, nuts, fresh caught fish, wild meat, or farm raised meat. There were no pesticides, herbicides, hormones or steroids used and our food was not chemically or genetically modified to triple the growth of our produce and meats. Food was for fuel and celebration. Throughout history there have been times when food was scarce which helped prevent the overindulgence we often see today.

I am not saying we should not enjoy food. What I am saying is let food be fuel most of the time and choose times to celebrate with food. Holidays, birthdays, anniversaries, and major milestones are good times to celebrate. Learning to balance how you consume food is so important. Be grateful for what has been prepared. God created our bodies to allow the digestive system to start producing enzymes that break down our food by just being grateful or smelling our food. These two actions: smelling and being grateful, will make you begin to salivate. In our saliva we have amylase. Amylase is an enzyme that breaks down carbohydrates and is an important part of the digestive process. Start practicing balance. Smell your food and be grateful at each meal. Fuel your body with the best possible food to help your body to begin to heal itself. Balance is key in all we do. Too much of anything, or not enough of some things, will create an unhealthy temple for the Holy Spirit.

Now over the next ninety days we are going to begin to clean up our diet. Each day begin looking at food as fuel. How do you want to feel? Do you want to be energetic? Do you want to recover from a workout faster? Do you want to sleep better? All these answers and more should be YES, YES, YES!!!!!! The way to do that is what you put into your body. Hence, food is fuel.

Each time you go to the grocery store stop buying processed foods. What are processed foods? Well, I was once told by my chiropractor "if it is grown on a plant and not made in a plant you can eat it". Basically, there is not a twinkie tree or a chip tree. If a food has been modified, broken down and fried do not eat it. Pasta is a processed food. Instant rice, instant oatmeal, and grits are processed foods. Crackers, cookies, cakes are processed foods. This will take time to learn and put together. Making new habits takes three weeks. Keeping the habits takes three months. This is one reason of the reasons why this is a ninety-day journal.

Take these ninety days to begin switching unclean foods for clean foods. Start journalling what you eat. Journalling is important! This is one way you can watch how your body responds to the foods you eat. Do you get tired after eating certain foods? Do you feel heavy or have digestive distress after eating certain foods? Do you have more energy? Are you sleeping better? Track all these things so you can judge what you should eat and what you should begin to eliminate. Typically, when you are eating clean and feel negative symptoms you may have food sensitivities or be allergic to certain foods.

Next, drinking pure water is essential. This does not include water enhancers. Chemical powders you put in your water to make it taste better. They are marketed to you to help increase energy, provide you with amino acids, or even increase protein and electrolytes. These water "enhancers" are not needed at this point in your journey. This does not include tea or coffee.

Drink a minimum of eight 8-ounce glasses of water. Drinking up to a gallon of water a day is optimal. We need the water to flush out the toxins and move our digestive system. Did you know our bodies are made up of mostly water? If we are dehydrated, we cannot reproduce healthy cells. Therefore, our immune system lowers, and our body begins to decay, also known as cancer. Our organs cannot regenerate without proper amounts of water which can lead to diabetes, auto immune disorders, high blood pressure, cardiovascular disease and the list can go on.

Supplements can also be of key importance. If you choose to use supplements, I recommend you research not only what is in the product, but where it comes from. Is the company transparent? Do they use certified organic products? Will they allow you to come to the farms or plants where they are grown or produced? These are important questions that may require important answers. Do not waste your money on products or supplements that will do more harm. Also, since I am not a doctor, I recommend you consult your doctor, and get blood work as soon as you can. See where your body levels are. Vitamins, thyroid, cortisol, glucose; this information will help you make a much wiser choice or decision regarding the supplements your body may need. Again, I recommend going as natural as you can with supplements, as well.

MOVEMENT

IF YOU ARE reading this journal and are already in great shape, moving and grooving on a regular basis, that is wonderful! However, this journal can help you in other aspects or even help you realize you could be out of balance in this area as well.

Jesus told us in the Bible to go out into the world and teach the Gospel. Well at that time there was no internet, no google, no social media, and no email. People had to get up, go out, and tell the story. People had to get up, go out, and collect food and water for the day. People had to move to take care of day-to-day needs. Jesus wanted us to move. I understand we are in a different day and age; however, that does not give us an out to not move. WE MUST MOVE!!!!

Our bodies were created to move. Our circulatory system has a pump. It is an organ called the heart. The heart has veins and arteries that move our blood throughout the body. That is great until the heart is not able to function because the body is not moving to exercise it. Your heart is an organ and a muscle. The heart needs to be exercised for the muscle to stay in top condition. Movement is important! There is also the lymphatic system. Guess what? The lymphatic system does not have a pump! Let me say that again, the lymphatic system does not have a pump. So, the fluid that is filtered out of the blood containing debris and toxins goes into the lymphatic system and is stored in the lymphatic fluid. The only way to filter and move this fluid through and out of the body is by moving! If you get sick easy, if a simple cold turns into a major health issue, then look at how much you move.

During the next ninety days we are going from the couch to a daily movement. Each day you will have an activity that you can do at home or in a gym. You will have no excuse not to move. You say I cannot get out of my chair and walk to the kitchen. There is no excuse. You can move! Decide to start moving and start simple. I will give you recommendations on most beginners' levels over the next ninety days. It is time to go out into the world and teach the gospel of Christ! Go to places to be an example of how God has walked with you each day to a healthier life. Be the witness that He intended you to be.

HOW TO CLEAN UP, PREPARE, AND GROW YOUR TEMPLE

LET ME SAY that God will meet you where you are! You may have been working out for a long time or you could be stuck on the couch. You may read the Bible daily or you may not even own one. You could have what appears to be a nice body but be physically, emotionally, or spiritually sick on the inside. This book is about healing the whole you. You are the temple in which the Holy Spirit resides, and God is absolutely ready to meet you right where you are.

- The first part of your daily journal will be for spiritual growth. You cannot grow spiritually without connecting with God, His Word, Jesus, and the Holy Spirit.
- Each day you will have a devotion. Once you read the daily devotion take time to meditate on how this resonates in your life. Write down in the space provided how you feel about what you just read. Do you need to change something in your life? Did this devotion hit a nerve?
- If you have prayer requests, write them as well.
- You will also list 3 things each day in which you are grateful. Some days you may repeat the same thing. This will begin to change as you grow in your faith.
- The second part of your daily journal is for nutrition. Your body cannot heal itself if you are not fueling it with what it needs or if you are fueling it with junk.
- Over the next few pages, you will learn how you should be eating for next ninety days. You will write down everything you eat. I get asked all the time why. Because writing it down holds you accountable. Writing it downs reminds you of what you have had to eat that day and will help you gauge how much you need to eat.
- When you begin to see your body change in a positive direction you will have a guide in which to return. You will be able to gauge which weeks you did best and where you need improvement.
- What foods you may be sensitive to and what foods made you lose weight faster. I suggest you write down notes on how your body responds before and after you eat. Are you hungrier one day and not as much a day later. Did that meal cause you to bloat? Did your skin begin to break out or is your complexion getting clearer. This information is extremely important to make note of.
- *The last part of your daily journal is for movement. You must move to live!
- The first 30 days there will be an exercise example. You can either do this or your own.
- The last 60 days you will create your daily movement using exercises In the movement section of the book. You must journal your workouts as well. What you did, and how long. If doing a High Intensity Interval Training (HIIT) write down what exercises, how long for each exercise, how long the rest between exercises and how many cycles.
- If you are lifting weights, you will put the exercise, the weight used, how many sets with how many repetitions.
- When you do cardio workouts put down the exercise and how long. (Examples: walking 30 minutes, biking 8 miles, kick boxing 45 minutes.)

- Also, you will need to note how you feel during and after your workouts. Did you get dizzy or weak? Were you energetic? Were you sore from a previous day's work out?
- Below is a place to log your measurements and weight.
- Do not weigh yourself daily. I suggest once a week or better once a month.
- Every 4 weeks take your measurements. In the notes write down when you begin to feel your cloths getting looser.

The more notes you write in the food and movement portion the better your lifestyle change will be. This is a foundation to the rest of the year and the rest of your life. You will be able to see what your body needs. Not what is best for your friends' body, but what is best for yours. We are all beautiful snowflakes. No one is alike. Our DNA is different and makes us perform differently.

Measurements:

Day 1　Day 30　Day 60　Day 90

Neck _____ _____ _____ _____

Chest _____ _____ _____ _____

Hips _____ _____ _____ _____

Right Bicep _____ _____ _____ _____

Right Thigh _____ _____ _____ _____

Right Calve _____ _____ _____ _____

Weight _____ _____ _____ _____

Food

MAKE A LIST of eating habits you should change. Examples: Sugar intake, processed foods, soft drinks, overeating, alcohol, eating too much dairy, don't drink enough water.

Each week take one of the habits and focus on that. Then the next continue working on that habit and add another. This is not a sprint; it is a marathon. We cannot change our lifestyle overnight.

Food Intake Recommendation

- Eat a protein and vegetable at every meal.
- Eat a snack meal 30 minutes before movement.
- Women eat minimum 90 grams of protein a day. Men eat minimum 120 grams of protein a day.
- Eat at least 4 to 6 servings of vegetables a day. (Raw, steamed or roasted)
- Eat 2 servings of fruit a day.
- Eat your fruit before 1:00pm. Choose low glycemic fruits examples: Berries or Granny Smith apples.
- Eat when you first become hungry, do not wait until you are starving. This is when we overeat. Try to keep your meals scheduled at the same time each day.

Processed foods should be one of your first habits to eliminate, then the process of eliminating sugar. These two foods cause you to crave other foods. Elimination will be difficult at first, please push through. If you have a headache, I recommend Himalayan salt under your tongue. By eating less processed food your sodium intake will lower, causing electrolyte imbalance. A little pink salt typically helps balance this, releasing a headache or eliminating dizzy spells or brain fog.

Remember these first ninety days are about practice. Changing your diet and movement is a strong mental change. Do not get overwhelmed or down on yourself. When you feel these emotions, regroup, and remember you can do all things through Christ who strengthens you.

Movement

(I want to stress again before you begin any physical activity consult your doctor.)

THIS IS THE part of the lifestyle that can be most difficult. Some may say I cannot get out of a chair. I am not able to walk. That is ok. If you can move your legs in the chair, that is where you begin. If you can move your arms in a chair, that is where you begin. If you can only move for 5 minutes that is where you begin. The thing is **BEGIN**. Do not be still any longer. You purchased this book to begin your journey; therefore, **BEGIN**.

You move at your pace not your friends. Your commitment is what will lead you to start each morning in prayer, eating healthier, and moving.

There are different levels of fitness you could be in. Let's call them groups for this purpose.

Group one: people not able to get out of a chair. This group can move arms or legs.

Legs	Arms
Flutter Kick Lift your legs up and down	Arm Circles Big
March in your chair	Arm Circles Small
Point and flex your feet	Bicep Curls
Scissors Kick your legs	Bicep Hammer Curls
Sit-down – Stand-up	Shoulder Press
	Triceps Kickbacks

Cardio
Cardio Drum: (Laundry Basket, Yoga Ball and Drumsticks)
Put your favorite upbeat music on and play the drums for as many songs as you can.
Air punch: 20 secs on 10 secs off as many times as you can

HIIT (High Intense Interval Training)

> Choose any 5 exercises above and go as fast as you can for 20 seconds on and 20 seconds off. Go through all 5 exercises and rest 1 minute then repeat 2-3 times.

Group two: this group cannot walk far or may have many physical disabilities.

Again, you are starting this journey where you are. If you can stand up and sit down that is an exercise if you repeat it for 20-30 seconds in a row, then rest and repeat. If you can only walk 5-10 minutes begin there.

Examples for people beginning with physical disabilities.

Cardio

Walking- begin walking as long as you are able. Then each day you walk that long. After a week walk a minute or two longer until you can walk 30 minutes. Once you can walk 30 minutes begin picking up your pace to walk further in the same amount of time.

HIIT

Choose 5 exercises below and do as fast as you can for 20-30 seconds on and 20 seconds off. Go through all five exercises and rest 1 minute. Then repeat 2-3 times.

Air Punching (standing or sitting) Knee Raises	Calf Raises
Arm Circles Big Forward	Single Leg Raises (laying on your back)
Arm Circles Big Backward	Sit and March
Arm Circles Small Backward	Sitting Flutter Kicks
Arm Circles Small Forward	Sitting Scissor Kicks
Bend and Touch Toes	Stand-up Sit-down
Bicep Curls Step Up & Down (on low step)	Wall Planks
Bicep Kickbacks	Wall Sits
Bridge Thrust Wall Push Up	

Do not begin lifting days until you are comfortable with cardio and HIIT. This should be around 30-45 days into the 90 days if you are consistent with food and movement. Again, I want you to push yourself to a positive desired burn. If you feel pain stop and reassess the exercise.

Group Three: this group may be able to walk, run, lift, and kick. You may have been an athlete in your younger years and just let life take over or you may be working out daily and want a new change. Whever you are in your fitness journey this book will provide examples that can challenge your current state of fitness; however, it is also a commitment between you and God to begin taking full responsibility of your temple with Him. Allow God to guide you in your daily life by putting Him first. I suggest alternating Cardio, HIIT and Strength Training. Begin where you are. If you are working out with a friend push each other but do not harm each other. Don't push to pain just push to burn.

Exercise Examples

CARDIO (Do cardio 30-45 minutes on cardio days.)	
Bike	Run
Cardio Drum	Walk
Kick Boxing	Walk-Run

HIIT

Pick 5-8 exercises below to create a cycle. Do each exercise as hard as you can for 30-60 seconds resting 20 seconds between exercises. After a complete cycle rest 1 minute. Repeat 2-4 times.

Knee Highs	Pikes	Inch Worms
Jumping Jacks	V-Push	Squat Jumps
Push Ups	V-Sit	Burpees
Jumping Jack	Planks	Wall Sits
Run in Place	Box Jumps	Skaters
Flip Tires	Bridge Thrust	Mountain Climbers
Ropes	Mummy Kicks	Air Punching
Slam Ball	Shoulder Kicks	

LIFTING	
Upper Body:	
Bicep Curls Close Grip	Lat Pull Down
Bicep Curls Wide Grip	Seated Row
Hammer Curls	Upright Row
Angle Bicep Curls	Bent Over Row
Triceps Pull Down	Shoulder Press
Triceps Kickback	Front arm Lift
Dips	Lateral Raise Lift
Overhead Triceps Extension	Incline Chest Press
Skull Crushers	Close Grip Chest Press
Single Overhead Angle Triceps Extension	Chest Press

Lower Body:	
Bridge Thrust	Plie' (Plee ay) Squats
Front Lunges	Side Lunges
Hip Thrust	Squats
Leg Curls	Walking Lunges
Leg Extensions	

LETS BEGIN

Holy Spirit Guide us Each Day!

Day 1

Date: _____

Matthew 17:20 (NIV)

He replied, "Because you have so little faith. Truly I tell you, if you have faith as small as a mustard seed, you can say to this mountain, 'Move from here to there,' and it will move. Nothing will be impossible for you."

GOD IS SO big, and we try to put him into a little box. We tuck this box away until we need to rub the little box for a wish to be granted. I am learning to throw the box away. I am trusting and walking each day asking, what will today bring? Will you send me people to talk to? Who needs you God? Help me lay myself down to serve you Father. Laying myself down is my way of asking Him to fill my temple and move me. Let me be the mountain He moves each day. Enable me to help people and encourage those who feel hopeless.

Today KNOW this: God is real, God can move mountains, God can heal, and God can FREE YOU!

What are you grateful for?

_____
_____
_____

Prayer Request

_____
_____
_____

What is keeping God in a box?

_____
_____
_____

What do you need to lay down today? How are you trying to put God into a box?

_____
_____
_____

Food Journal	Movement
Water _ _ _ _ _ _ _ _ _ _ _ _ _	**Cardio** 30 minutes
	What Type:

Meal 1	Time:	How do you feel before?
Protein		
Fruit		
Vegetable		
Fat		

Meal 2	Time:	How do you feel during?
Protein		
Fruit		
Vegetable		
Fat		

Meal 3	Time:	How do you feel after?
Protein		
Fruit		
Vegetable		
Fat		

Snack	Time:	
Protein		
Vegetable		

Day 2

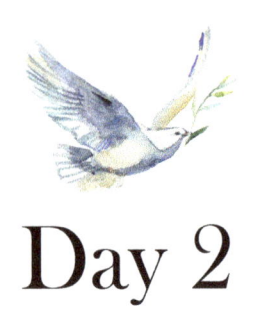

Date: _____

1 Corinthians 13:11 (NIV)
When I was a child, I spoke like a child, I thought like a child, I reasoned like a child.
When I became a man, I put the ways of childhood behind me.

YES, GOD WANTS us to grow. He tells us here we need to put away childish things. However, I believe we must still possess a childlike faith as we grow in our boldness and understanding of God.

He wants us to have all of Him and lean on Him when we are weak. We should lift others when we are in our stronger times with His word.

Take time each day to grow stronger in the Word. Meditate on Him each day so you can hear and feel His guidance.

What are you grateful for?

_____
_____
_____

Prayer Request

_____
_____
_____

What are you dealing with as a child today?

_____
_____
_____

Where can you grow in your daily walk today?

_____
_____
_____

Food Journal		Movement
Water _ _ _ _ _ _ _ _ _ _ _		**HIIT**
Meal 1	Time:	Bicycle Crunches
Protein		Jumping Jacks
		Knee Highs
Fruit		Plank
Vegetable		Pike Ab Exercise
Fat		

Meal 2	Time:	How do you feel before?
Protein		
Fruit		
Vegetable		
Fat		

Meal 3	Time:	How do you feel during?
Protein		
Fruit		
Vegetable		
Fat		

Snack	Time:	How do you feel after?
Protein		
Vegetable		

Day 3

Date: _____

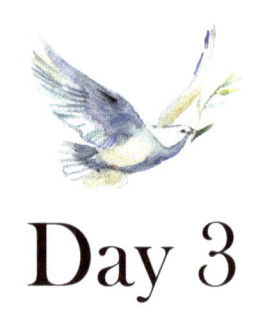

1 Corinthians 16:13-14 (NIV)
Be on your guard; stand firm in the faith; be courageous; be strong.
Do everything in love.

EACH DAY WE should put our armor on and pray God will keep us through the day. Help us to be the warriors You created.

We must love!

Love can heal – Love can pick another up – Love can make your day better.

So today armor up and love!

What are you grateful for?

_____
_____
_____

Prayer Request

_____
_____
_____

What have you been wavering on?

_____
_____
_____

How can you change what you wrote above through God?

_____
_____
_____

Food Journal		Movement
Water _ _ _ _ _ _ _ _ _ _ _ _		**Upper Body:**
Meal 1	Time:	Bicep Curls
Protein		Wide Grip Bicep Curls
		Overhead Triceps Extensions
Fruit		Triceps Kick Back
Vegetable		Plank
Fat		

Meal 2	Time:	How do you feel before?
Protein		
Fruit		
Vegetable		
Fat		

Meal 3	Time:	How do you feel during?
Protein		
Fruit		
Vegetable		
Fat		

Snack	Time:	How do you feel after?
Protein		
Vegetable		

Day 4

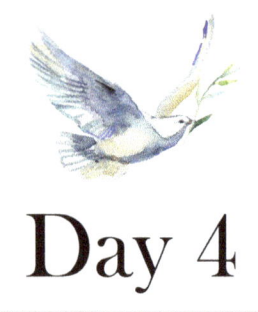

Date: _____

Matthew 18:2-4 (NIV)

2 He called a little child to him and placed the child among them. 3 And he said: "Truly I tell you, unless you change and become like little children, you will never enter the kingdom of heaven. 4 Therefore, whoever takes the lowly position of this child is the greatest in the kingdom of heaven.

DO YOU REALIZE that a childlike faith is almost a superpower? We allow so many things to change our minds, to create fear and move us in the wrong direction. If we just stop, breathe, and let God take control we will see a better outcome. Children have faith that God will do just that. Nothing has tainted their minds to think any other way.

Today blow bubbles and sing a song from your childhood. Allow yourself to be in the childlike manner so you can remember what it is like to let go and let God.

What are you grateful for?

_____
_____
_____

Prayer Request

_____
_____
_____

Why do you feel like you have to be the leader in your life? Why will you not allow God to take control?

_____
_____
_____
_____

Food Journal	**Movement**
Water __ __ __ __ __ __ __ __ __ __	**Cardio** 30 minutes
	What Type:

Meal 1	Time:	How do you feel before?
Protein		
Fruit		
Vegetable		
Fat		

Meal 2	Time:	How do you feel during?
Protein		
Fruit		
Vegetable		
Fat		

Meal 3	Time:	How do you feel after?
Protein		
Fruit		
Vegetable		
Fat		

Snack	Time:
Protein	
Vegetable	

Day 5

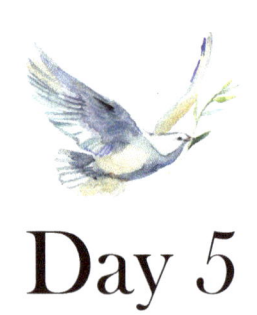

Date: _____

<u>Luke 8:25 (NIV)</u>

"Where is your faith?" he asked his disciples. In fear and amazement, they asked one another, "Who is this? He commands even the winds and the water, and they obey him."

Faith: Believing in something you cannot see.

RIDING OUT A physical storm. Sometimes we have storms in our lives that may not be physical but are mental. Our human mind does not know how to get through them. We need to pray and seek God during these times. Stand and know God is with us. We must allow our Faith in God help us ride out the storm.

Next time you see a friend that is causing drama, sit and lean on God. When anxiety is rising, get on your knees and praise God.

These storms will pass, and He will get the Glory. Do not react in fear or worldly ways. God is always there, reach out your hand and allow God to take the lead.

What are you grateful for?

_____
_____
_____

Prayer Request

_____
_____
_____

What storms are you riding today? Are people getting in the way of what you desire? Do you allow others to dictate how you spend your time? Do you have fears that you need to lay at the feet of Jesus?

_____
_____
_____

Food Journal		Movement
Water _ _ _ _ _ _ _ _ _ _		**HIIT**
Meal 1	Time:	Mummy Kicks
Protein		Air Punches
		Wall sit
Fruit		Scissor Kicks (Ab exercise)
Vegetable		Plank
Fat		

Meal 2	Time:	How do you feel before?
Protein		
Fruit		
Vegetable		
Fat		

Meal 3	Time:	How do you feel during?
Protein		
Fruit		
Vegetable		
Fat		

Snack	Time:	How do you feel after?
Protein		
Vegetable		

Day 6

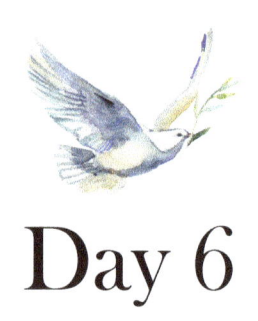

Date: _____

2 Corinthians 10:5 (NIV)
We demolish arguments and every pretension that sets itself up against the knowledge of God, and we take captive every thought to make it obedient to Christ.

ON OCTOBER 3, 2022, I was called to be baptized. This time not as a proclamation of my faith in new acceptance of Jesus Christ, but to be obedient in washing away all that I have allowed to happen in my life. It was time to rise cleansed as a new being.

This does not mean I will be perfect. This does not mean I will not fall short. This means on October 3, 2022, I made a stand to be obedient to what God is calling me to do each day. I will take my thoughts captive. I will walk in His Word and treat my temple with respect.

Today keep your mind on Him. When someone is not in line with your heart give it to God. Don't allow the negativity of satan to move you out of the path God has for you. Today put on His Word and walk in faith and courage.

What are you grateful for?

_____
_____
_____

Prayer Request

_____
_____
_____

What are you allowing to get in Gods way? Where are you not being obedient?

_____
_____
_____

Food Journal		Movement
Water _ _ _ _ _ _ _ _ _ _ _ _		**Lower Body:**
Meal 1	Time:	Bridge Thrust
Protein		Calf Raises
Fruit		Side to Side Lunges
Vegetable		Squats
Fat		Step Ups

Meal 2	Time:	How do you feel before?
Protein		
Fruit		
Vegetable		
Fat		

Meal 3	Time:	How do you feel during?
Protein		
Fruit		
Vegetable		
Fat		

Snack	Time:	How do you feel after?
Protein		
Vegetable		

Day 7

Date: _____

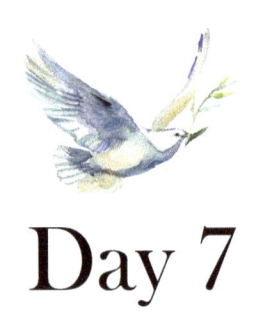

Proverbs 4:23 (NIV)
Above all else, guard your heart, for everything you do flows from it.

TODAY MAKE SURE your thoughts are of good and pure nature. If your thoughts are not pure take them to God. Find the root of the negativity and allow Him to take it from you.

Your thoughts become actions! Let that sink in today! Meditate on how God wants to change your thought processes.

What are you grateful for?

_____
_____
_____

Prayer Request

_____
_____
_____

What are the most difficult thoughts you have a hard time taking captive? Where do these thoughts stem from?

_____
_____
_____
_____
_____

Food Journal		Movement
Water _ _ _ _ _ _ _ _ _ _ _ _ _		Rest Day
		You can do Active Rest

Meal 1	Time:	
Protein		Walk at a slow pace.
Fruit		Low impact hiking
Vegetable		Low impact biking
Fat		

Meal 2	Time:	How do you feel before?
Protein		
Fruit		
Vegetable		
Fat		

Meal 3	Time:	How do you feel during?
Protein		
Fruit		
Vegetable		
Fat		

Snack	Time:	How do you feel after?
Protein		
Vegetable		

Day 8

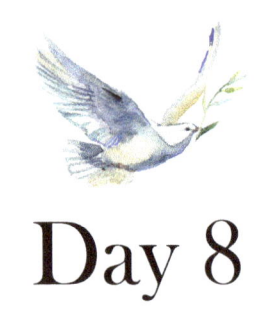

Date: _____

Matthew 15:18 (NIV)
But the things that come out of a person's mouth come from the heart, and these defile them.

OUR MINDS ARE so powerful and can make or break a person. When we think negatively, we do not have our mind and heart on the purpose of God. When we are not walking in the Word and prayer, we walk in the world and on our own volition. This is when we see ourselves making the wrong decisions, and we find our lives full of drama.

Looking back through the past few days, think about what choices you have made. Were you beginning your day in the word and prayer? Did the choices you made bring peace and joy, or did drama, and negativity evolve?

_____
_____
_____

What are you grateful for?

_____
_____
_____

Prayer Request

_____
_____
_____

Food Journal	Movement
Water _ _ _ _ _ _ _ _ _ _ _	**Cardio** 30 minutes
	What Type:

Meal 1	Time:	How do you feel before?
Protein		
Fruit		
Vegetable		
Fat		

Meal 2	Time:	How do you feel during?
Protein		
Fruit		
Vegetable		
Fat		

Meal 3	Time:	How do you feel after?
Protein		
Fruit		
Vegetable		
Fat		

Snack	Time:
Protein	
Vegetable	

Day 9

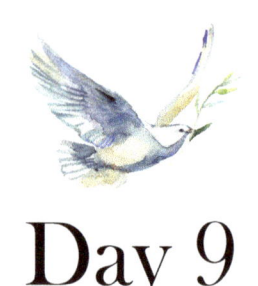

Date: _____

Psalms 118
Read the whole chapter.

LAST NIGHT MY daughter called me and told me about her day. She didn't feel she was treated fairly at work, and the situation was not handled in private.
My first reaction was to love her.
My second reaction was to protect her.
My third reaction was to guide her.
Reflecting over our conversation I felt God was telling me this is how He wants to treat His children as well.
Love-Protect-Guide
Know His mercy and grace.
Know He will protect you against the things of this world.
We cannot control others' thoughts or actions, but we can control our own thoughts and actions.
Lean into God, allowing him to guide you and teach you how to handle daily situations.

What do you do when you have a tough decision to make? How do you respond when you feel treated unfairly?

_____
_____
_____

What are you grateful for?

_____
_____
_____

Prayer Request

_____
_____
_____

What have you been wavering on?

_____
_____
_____

Food Journal			Movement	
Water __ __ __ __ __ __ __ __ __ __			**HIIT**	
Meal 1	Time:		Mountain Climbers	
Protein			Side Plank Left	
			Side Plank Right	
Fruit			Dips	
Vegetable			Push Ups (if on your knees do not lift your feet off the ground)	
Fat				

Meal 2	Time:	How do you feel before?
Protein		
Fruit		
Vegetable		
Fat		

Meal 3	Time:	How do you feel during?
Protein		
Fruit		
Vegetable		
Fat		

Snack	Time:	How do you feel after?
Protein		
Vegetable		

Day 10

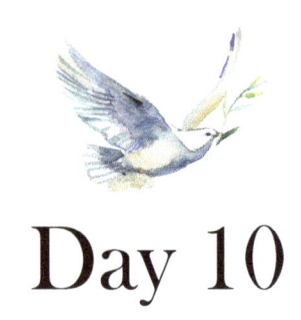

Date: _____

1 Corinthians 10:31 (NIV)

So, whether you eat or drink or whatever you do, do it all for the glory of God.

THERE ARE NO quick fixes in health. No miracle pills to transform your body in a week. We need to look at ourselves and be honest. Did it take a day or a week to get to the point where you feel you are not liking what you see or feel the way you feel?

This is what you need to look at:

What are you eating?
What are you drinking?
What pharmaceuticals are you putting into your body?
Are you moving?
Do you eat, drink, and move in ways that will heal your body?
Do you supplement your body with elements that heal or destroy your body?

On the 3rd day of creation, God made everything we need to heal our bodies.

Today, think about what you are doing to fuel your body. What can you change?

_____
_____
_____

What are you grateful for?

_____
_____
_____

Prayer Request

_____
_____
_____

Food Journal		Movement
Water _ _ _ _ _ _ _ _ _ _ _ _		**Upper Body:**
Meal 1	Time:	Front Arm Raises
Protein		Side Arm Raises
		Should Press
Fruit		Bent over Rows
Vegetable		Seated Row
Fat		

Meal 2	Time:	How do you feel before?
Protein		
Fruit		
Vegetable		
Fat		

Meal 3	Time:	How do you feel during?
Protein		
Fruit		
Vegetable		
Fat		

Snack	Time:	How do you feel after?
Protein		
Vegetable		

Day 11

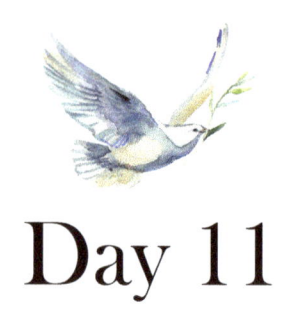

Date: _____

1 Thessalonians 5:18 (NIV)
Give thanks in all circumstances; for this is God's will for you in Christ Jesus.

WHEN YOU WAKE and realize you are breathing, give thanks. When you have a coffee or breakfast, give thanks. If your family is still in reach by touch or phone, give thanks. There is so much in which to be grateful. Don't save it up for one day of the year. Each day tell God what you are grateful for. In these moments you are strengthened. When you are giving thanks there is no room in your mind and heart for negativity. WOW!! What a powerful thought process.

Today give thanks all day! Every second you can give thanks.

STOP THE NEGATIVITY.

What are negative thoughts you need to release? What can you replace them with?

_____
_____
_____

What are you grateful for?

_____
_____
_____

Prayer Request

_____
_____
_____

Food Journal	**Movement**
Water _ _ _ _ _ _ _ _ _ _ _ _ _ _	**Cardio** 30 minutes
	What Type:

Meal 1	Time:	How do you feel before?
Protein		
Fruit		
Vegetable		
Fat		

Meal 2	Time:	How do you feel during
Protein		
Fruit		
Vegetable		
Fat		

Meal 3	Time:	How do you feel after?
Protein		
Fruit		
Vegetable		
Fat		

Snack	Time:	
Protein		
Vegetable		

Day 12

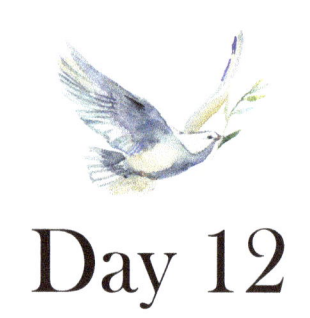

Date: _____

Jeremiah 29:11 (NIV)
For I know the plans I have for you," declares the LORD, "plans to prosper you and not to harm you, plans to give you hope and a future.

.

GOD WANTED THE best for you since the day you took your first breath. Why then do we as humans want to go against His wishes?

Why do we allow the things of this world to move us instead of allowing our creator to move us?

All God wants is our time, and for us to be whole. He wants us to live in a place of peace, joy, and most of all Love.

Today, think about this: What are you allowing to move you instead of God? Why are you not allowing God to move in you during these times?

_____
_____
_____

What are you grateful for?

_____
_____
_____

Prayer Request

_____
_____
_____

Food Journal		Movement
Water _ _ _ _ _ _ _ _ _ _		**HIIT**
Meal 1	Time:	Mountain Climbers
Protein		Side Plank Left
		Side Plank Right
Fruit		Dips
Vegetable		Push Ups (if on your knees do not lift your feet off the ground)
Fat		

Meal 2	Time:	How do you feel before?
Protein		
Fruit		
Vegetable		
Fat		

Meal 3	Time:	How do you feel during?
Protein		
Fruit		
Vegetable		
Fat		

Snack	Time:	How do you feel after?
Protein		
Vegetable		

Day 13

Date: _____

Proverbs 15:1 (NIV)
A gentle answer turns away wrath, but a harsh word stirs up anger.

Thinking about my insides today:
Am I humble?
Am I kind?
Am I edifying?
If I think about how I speak to others, I can answer those questions.

GOD CALLS US to be gentle when dealing with people, even if they are not so gentle with us. Our words can cut like a knife. Even if the world tells us that is a good thing, we do not feel so good afterwards if we succumb to the world.
If our hearts are lined up with God and we are seeking His will then our tongue should be gentle.

Take inventory today. Think of the questions above. How can you change?

_____
_____
_____
_____

What are you grateful for?

_____
_____
_____

Prayer Request

_____
_____
_____

Food Journal		Movement
Water _ _ _ _ _ _ _ _ _ _ _ _ _ _ _		Lower Body:
Meal 1	Time:	Bridge Thrust
Protein		Calf Raises
Fruit		Side to Side Lunges
Vegetable		Squats
		Step Ups
Fat		

Meal 2	Time:	How do you feel before?
Protein		
Fruit		
Vegetable		
Fat		

Meal 3	Time:	How do you feel during?
Protein		
Fruit		
Vegetable		
Fat		

Snack	Time:	How do you feel after?
Protein		
Vegetable		

Day 14

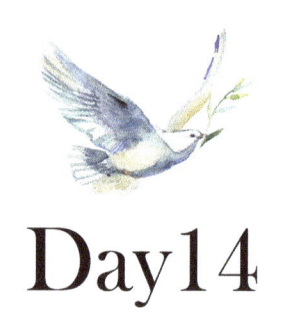

Date: _____

Exodus 24:7 (NIV)
Then he took the Book of the Covenant and read it to the people. They responded, "We will do everything the LORD has said; we will obey."

Are you being obedient?

Do you know what obedience is?

Obedience is doing what you are told.

How do we know we are doing what God tells us?

FIRST, HE SAYS to read the word daily. His Word is our "Playbook", instruction manual if you will.

If we are not reading the word daily, we will not know what we need to do to be obedient.

If you are not reading the Word daily, I challenge you to read daily. Then ask God to show you the steps to obedience.

What are you grateful for?

_____
_____
_____

Prayer Request

_____
_____
_____

Food Journal	Movement
Water _ _ _ _ _ _ _ _ _ _ _ _	Rest Day
	You can do Active Rest

Meal 1	Time:	
Protein		Walk at a slow pace.
Fruit		Low impact hiking
Vegetable		Low impact biking
Fat		

Meal 2	Time:	How do you feel before?
Protein		
Fruit		
Vegetable		
Fat		

Meal 3	Time:	How do you feel during?
Protein		
Fruit		
Vegetable		
Fat		

Snack	Time:	How do you feel after?
Protein		
Vegetable		

Day 15

Date: _____

Mark 6:34 (NIV)
When Jesus landed and saw a large crowd, he had compassion on them, because they were like sheep without a shepherd. So, he began teaching them many things.

I SPEAK A lot about moving our bodies, but what about when we are moved emotionally? God will move you in many ways. He will speak to you in many ways. Jesus was moved with compassion.

Start today getting closer to God so you can hear Him and feel Him when He is moving in you.

Be ready to move emotionally and physically when you are called on by God?

Have you heard or felt God moving in your life? List ways you have heard or felt His presence or calling.

_____
_____
_____

What are you grateful for?

_____
_____
_____

Prayer Request

_____
_____
_____

Food Journal	Movement
Water __ __ __ __ __ __ __ __ __ __	**Cardio** 30 minutes
	What Type:

Meal 1	Time:	How do you feel before?
Protein		
Fruit		
Vegetable		
Fat		

Meal 2	Time:	How do you feel during?
Protein		
Fruit		
Vegetable		
Fat		

Meal 3	Time:	How do you feel after?
Protein		
Fruit		
Vegetable		
Fat		

Snack	Time:
Protein	
Vegetable	

Day 16

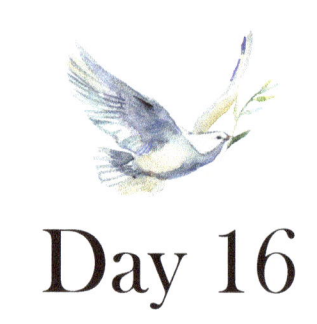

Date: _____

Philippians 4:8 (NIV)

Finally, brothers and sisters, whatever is true, whatever is noble, whatever is right, whatever is pure, whatever is lovely, whatever is admirable—if anything is excellent or praiseworthy—think about such things.

Here it is!

Here is what God wants us to think about all day every day!

Wash your mind in the word so you can continuously think of truth! Honesty! Purity! Love!

GOOD AND PURE THOUGHTS ALL DAY!

IF WE FILL our minds and hearts with these things, we do not have room for the evil and negativity that the world brings down and tries to destroy in us.

List positive thoughts you can use throughout the day that will reverse the negative thoughts you would normally think.

_____
_____
_____
_____

What are you grateful for?

_____
_____
_____

Prayer Request

_____
_____
_____

Food Journal		Movement
Water _ _ _ _ _ _ _ _ _ _		**HIIT**
Meal 1	Time:	Sprints
Protein		Air Punches
Fruit		Grass Grabbers
Vegetable		Knee Highs
Fat		V Push Ab exercise

Meal 2	Time:	How do you feel before?
Protein		
Fruit		
Vegetable		
Fat		

Meal 3	Time:	How do you feel during?
Protein		
Fruit		
Vegetable		
Fat		

Snack	Time:	How do you feel after?
Protein		
Vegetable		

Day 17

Date: _____

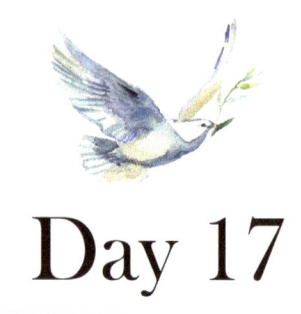

Psalms 62:8 (NIV)
Trust in him at all times, you people; pour out your hearts to him,
for God is our refuge.

GOD TELLS US to trust in Him at all times. When drama presents itself to us in life we need to stop, drop, and pray. Trust that God is already in route to help us. When we decide to take the oncoming drama into our own hands, we escalate the issue. God dissolves the issue.

When adversity comes your way don't automatically react. Take a moment to stop what you are doing and remove yourself. Sit still and pray. Begin to listen to how God wants you to respond.

Today, pray God will give you the courage to remove yourself and to seek His wisdom.

List times you reacted without seeking God's wisdom. Then think of how the issue could have played out if you removed yourself and allowed God to work.

___

What are you grateful for?

___

Prayer Request

___

Food Journal		Movement
Water _ _ _ _ _ _ _ _ _ _ _		**Lower Body:** 3 sets of 12 each exercise
Meal 1	Time:	Bridge Thrust
Protein		(after 12 reps hold at top 10 seconds)
Fruit		Donkey Kick Leg Raise L
		Donkey Kick Leg Raise R
Vegetable		Forward Lunge Lunge L
Fat		Forward Lunge Lunge R

Meal 2	Time:	How do you feel before?
Protein		
Fruit		
Vegetable		
Fat		

Meal 3	Time:	How do you feel during?
Protein		
Fruit		
Vegetable		
Fat		

Snack	Time:	How do you feel after?
Protein		
Vegetable		

Day 18

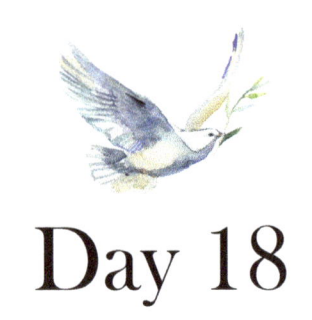

Date: _____

Psalms 145:18-21 (NIV)

18 The LORD is near to all who call on him, to all who call on him in truth.
19 He fulfills the desires of those who fear him; He hears their cry and saves them.
20 The LORD watches over all who love Him, but all the wicked he will destroy.
21 My mouth will speak in praise of the LORD. Let every creature praise
His holy name for ever and ever.

GOD WANTS TO be able to give you what you need and desire. We must seek Him and His purpose. In all that you do today seek Him. Walk in His wisdom.

What is it you are trying to do on your own that is not working for you?

_____
_____
_____

Have you prayed over this? Does it line up with the purpose God has given you?

What are you grateful for?

_____
_____
_____

Prayer Request

_____
_____
_____

Food Journal	Movement
Water __ __ __ __ __ __ __ __ __ __	**Cardio** 30 minutes
	What Type:

Meal 1	Time:	How do you feel before?
Protein		
Fruit		
Vegetable		
Fat		

Meal 2	Time:	How do you feel during?
Protein		
Fruit		
Vegetable		
Fat		

Meal 3	Time:	How do you feel during?
Protein		
Fruit		
Vegetable		
Fat		

Snack	Time:
Protein	
Vegetable	

Day 19

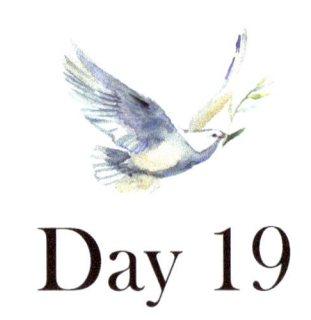

Date: _____

Isaiah 55:8-9 (NIV)

8 "For my thoughts are not your thoughts, neither are your ways my ways," declares the LORD. 9 "As the heavens are higher than the earth, so are my ways higher than your ways and my thoughts than your thoughts.

TODAY, FOCUS ON God. Do not focus on your work or your weekend, but what God desires for you. We get wrapped up in what we want and think as a human, but we do not spend time with God. Do we seek what His purpose is?

When we stop putting Him first our world falls apart. We become bitter, insecure, and depressed. When we seek God first joy returns, our minds clear, and we become focused. We love stronger.

What have you been wrestling with lately? How can you allow God to turn it around?

_____
_____
_____
_____

What are you grateful for?

_____
_____
_____

Prayer Request

_____
_____
_____

Food Journal		**Movement**
Water _ _ _ _ _ _ _ _ _ _ _ _ _ _		**HIIT**
Meal 1	Time:	Jump Rope
Protein		Plank Jacks
Fruit		Reverse Sit ups
Vegetable		Plank Taps
^		(alternate taping your shoulders)
Fat		Walking Lunges

Meal 2	Time:	How do you feel before?
Protein		
Fruit		
Vegetable		
Fat		

Meal 3	Time:	How do you feel during?
Protein		
Fruit		
Vegetable		
Fat		

Snack	Time:	How do you feel after?
Protein		
Vegetable		

Day 20

Date: _____

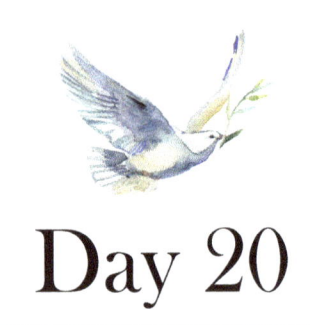

Ecclesiastes 3 Read the First Half of the Chapter

TO EVERYTHING THERE is a season. A time and purpose under the heavens.
God knew when He created the world we would mourn. He knew our world would flip upside down at times.
He gives us hope, joy, and love if we just seek it. We will get though the hard valleys and we will laugh and dance again.
Do not look at the valleys as punishment. Begin to look at these valleys as opportunities to be molded into the warrior you are becoming.

What valleys have you gone through lately? What strengths can you find that you did not realize you were gaining when you came through?

_____
_____
_____
_____

What are you grateful for?

_____
_____
_____

Prayer Request

_____
_____
_____

Food Journal		Movement
Water _ _ _ _ _ _ _ _ _ _ _ _		**Full Body:** 3 sets of 12 each exercise
Meal 1	Time:	Dips
Protein		Hammer Curls
Fruit		L Lifts (Front raise and side)
Vegetable		Leg Extension
Fat		Leg Curls

Meal 2	Time:	How do you feel before?
Protein		
Fruit		
Vegetable		
Fat		

Meal 3	Time:	How do you feel during?
Protein		
Fruit		
Vegetable		
Fat		

Snack	Time:	How do you feel after?
Protein		
Vegetable		

Day 21

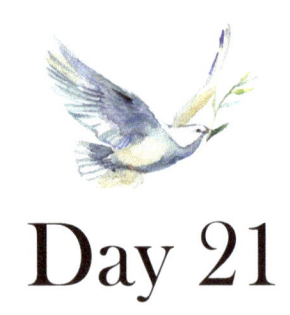

Date: _____

Ecclesiastes 3:6 (NIV)
A time to search and a time to give up, a time to keep and a time to throw away.

SOMETIMES WE ARE called to do things we do not understand. We may have to leave a place where we have lived or worked or worshiped. Maybe we need to be separated from lifelong friends.

Before you make a move or take a step, confirm it lines up with the word. Seek God's will in the situation until you have peace. God may move you or move people around you to accomplish things far greater than you could ever imagine.

Seek His purpose and will and He will meet you there.

Is there a difficult decision you are faced with? Does it line up with the word or the purpose you know God has for you? Don't make it more difficult than it needs to be.

What are you grateful for?

_____
_____
_____

Prayer Request

_____
_____
_____

Food Journal	Movement
Water _ _ _ _ _ _ _ _ _ _ _ _	**Rest Day**
	You can do Active Rest

Meal 1	Time:	
Protein		Walk at a slow pace.
Fruit		Low impact hiking
Vegetable		Low impact biking
Fat		

Meal 2	Time:	How do you feel before?
Protein		
Fruit		
Vegetable		
Fat		

Meal 3	Time:	How do you feel during?
Protein		
Fruit		
Vegetable		
Fat		

Snack	Time:	How do you feel after?
Protein		
Vegetable		

Day 22

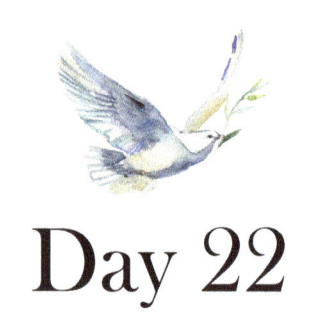

Date: _____

Deuteronomy 31:6 (NIV)
Be strong and courageous. Do not be afraid or terrified because of them, for the LORD your God goes with you; He will never leave you nor forsake you."

IF WE SET our eyes on the ways of the world fear can begin to grow in our hearts. This fear can then begin to take hold of our minds, and then show up in our actions. Today instead of allowing that to happen let's press into the Word and listen to God.

Be strong! Fear not! God is with you. This is the time to keep your eyes and ears on God and not the world. Seek him and find strength.

Today be strong, and list fear you want to let go to God.

_____
_____
_____

What are you grateful for?

_____
_____
_____

Prayer Request

_____
_____
_____

Food Journal	Movement
Water __ __ __ __ __ __ __ __ __ __	**Cardio** 30 minutes
	What Type:

Meal 1	Time:	How do you feel before?
Protein		
Fruit		
Vegetable		
Fat		

Meal 2	Time:	How do you feel during?
Protein		
Fruit		
Vegetable		
Fat		

Meal 3	Time:	How do you feel after?
Protein		
Fruit		
Vegetable		
Fat		

Snack	Time:
Protein	
Vegetable	

Day 23

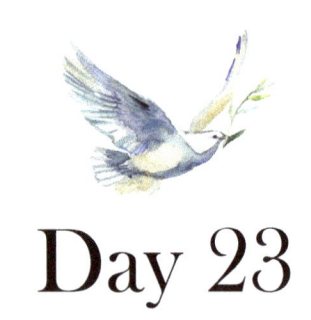

Date: _____

Psalms 32:8-9 (NIV)

8 I will instruct you and teach you in the way you should go; I will counsel you with my loving eyes on you. 9 Do not be like the horse or the mule, which have no understanding but must be controlled by bit and bridle or they will not come to you.

Why do we fight to get our way? Do we not realize that God has a better way? While I am spending more time with God, I am hearing Him clearer.

He says don't be a mule. Don't be so stubborn. Do you see the big mess you are making doing it your way? How many times have we decided to take issues into our own hands? We don't listen to what God wants to tell us or ask what He would do. I know when I have a problem, and I try to solve it on my own, it gets much worse.

TODAY SPEND TIME asking and listening to God before you make a step. Read the word so you know your actions line up with God's plan. Don't be a stubborn mule and see how much better your day will go.

List thing you are doing on your own, and how you are going to allow God to take over.

_____
_____
_____

What are you grateful for?

_____
_____
_____

Prayer Request

_____
_____
_____

Food Journal		Movement
Water _ _ _ _ _ _ _ _ _ _ _ _ _ _		**HIIT**
Meal 1	Time:	Jump Rope
Protein		Plank Jacks
		Reverse Sit ups
Fruit		Plank Taps
Vegetable		(alternate taping your shoulders)
Fat		Walking Lunges

Meal 2	Time:	How do you feel before?
Protein		
Fruit		
Vegetable		
Fat		

Meal 3	Time:	How do you feel during?
Protein		
Fruit		
Vegetable		
Fat		

Snack	Time:	How do you feel after?
Protein		
Vegetable		

Day 24

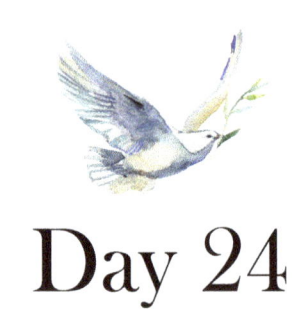

Date: _____

Romans 3:27-28 (NIV)

27 Where, then, is boasting? It is excluded. Because of what law? The law that requires works. No, because of the law that requires faith. 28 For we maintain that a person is justified by faith apart from the works of the law.

HOW MANY TIMES, pridefully, do we boast? How many times do we boast when we do something for others? How many times do we boast when God does an amazing thing?

We need to be humble and quiet. Let people see what is going on and not tell them sometimes. Learning to humble yourself is quite a difficult task for some people.

Where in your life do you need to humble yourself? How can God help you in these areas?

_____
_____
_____

What are you grateful for?

_____
_____
_____

Prayer Request

_____
_____
_____

Food Journal		Movement
Water _ _ _ _ _ _ _ _ _ _ _ _		**Upper Body:** 3 sets of 12 each exercise
Meal 1	Time:	Chest Press
Protein		Chest Flies
Fruit		Pull Ups (Use pull up assist machine. Wide grip then close)
Vegetable		Plank (up to 1 minute each set)
Fat		

Meal 2	Time:	How do you feel before?
Protein		
Fruit		
Vegetable		
Fat		

Meal 3	Time:	How do you feel during?
Protein		
Fruit		
Vegetable		
Fat		

Snack	Time:	How do you feel after?
Protein		
Vegetable		

Day 25

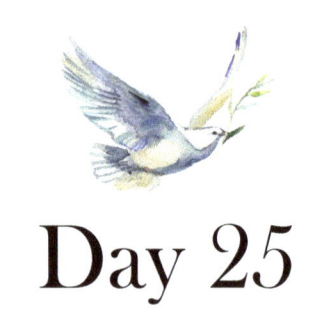

Date: _____

Isaiah 8:20 (NIV)

20 Consult God's instruction and the testimony of warning. If anyone does not speak according to this word, they have no light of dawn.

HAVE YOU EVER had something pop up and couldn't decide whether you should or should not do it? It is difficult to not be transformed by this Word. We want to do what our friends are doing. We walk through life thinking that if it feels good it must be good. Do the things you do, the thoughts you have, and the people you associate with line up with what the Word of God says. Do you know the word? Are you reading the word? Are you spending time with God to hear and feel the direction He is leading you? Seeking God each day may be difficult at first. Do what is difficult until it isn't.

Take a moment to reflect on your day when it is problematic and ask yourself, did you do it God's way or did you do it your way? We must daily walk and talk with God like he is our friend. Only then will we walk and talk in His direction and purpose.

Take inventory today of life steps you need to allow God to direct you. Are you listening to Him? Are you reading His Word daily?

_____
_____
_____

What are you grateful for?

_____
_____
_____

Prayer Request

_____
_____
_____

Food Journal		**Movement**
Water __ __ __ __ __ __ __ __ __ __		**Cardio** 30 minutes
		What Type:

Meal 1	Time:	How do you feel before?
Protein		
Fruit		
Vegetable		
Fat		

Meal 2	Time:	How do you feel during?
Protein		
Fruit		
Vegetable		
Fat		

Meal 3	Time:	How do you feel after?
Protein		
Fruit		
Vegetable		
Fat		

Snack	Time:
Protein	
Vegetable	

Day 26

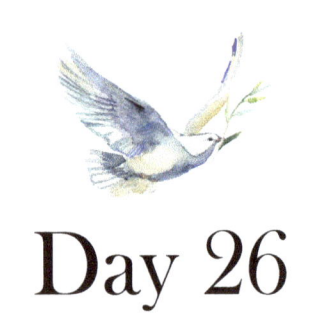

Date: _____

Mark 13:31 (NIV)

Heaven and earth will pass away, but my words will never pass away.

GOD'S WORDS ARE always with us. During hard and difficult days, He is always there. John 1:1 In the beginning was the Word and the Word was with God. God has always been and always will be.

When you are having a hard day remember you can lay your head down and know He is always nearby.

What are you struggling with today that you need God to hear?

_____
_____
_____

What are you grateful for?

_____
_____
_____

Prayer Request

_____
_____
_____

Food Journal		Movement
Water _ _ _ _ _ _ _ _ _ _ _ _		**Lower Body:** 3 sets of 12 each exercise
Meal 1	Time:	Alternating Step ups Calf Raises Leg Lifts Left 10 Right 10 Plie (Plee-ay) Squats Walking Lunges 10 up & back
Protein		
Fruit		
Vegetable		
Fat		

Meal 2	Time:	How do you feel before?
Protein		
Fruit		
Vegetable		
Fat		

Meal 3	Time:	How do you feel during?
Protein		
Fruit		
Vegetable		
Fat		

Snack	Time:	How do you feel after?
Protein		
Vegetable		

Day 27

Date: _____

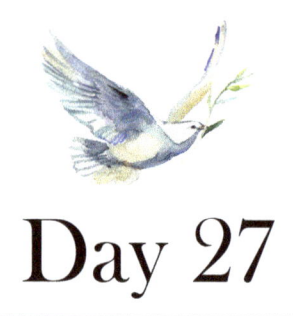

Exodus chapters 5-11

WE LEARN ABOUT Moses and the Israelites being in bondage and Moses setting them free. This was not an overnight process. The king of Egypt had a will of his own. We have our own free will to choose God and so does every person around us. So, if we are not seeing our promises today that does not mean God has not answered. Stand strong like Moses and Aaron, don't back down. If you are staying in the word, being diligent about keeping your faith and life lined up with God, then you and God will win.

Seek your strength from Him each day. Watch how you will grow.

What promises have you been waiting for?

_____
_____
_____

What are you grateful for?

_____
_____
_____

Prayer Request

_____
_____
_____

Food Journal		**Movement**
Water _ _ _ _ _ _ _ _ _ _ _		**HIIT**
Meal 1	Time:	Jumping Jacks
Protein		Reverse Sit Ups
		Soldier Kicks
Fruit		V Sit
Vegetable		Wall Sit with calf raises
Fat		

Meal 2	Time:	How do you feel before?
Protein		
Fruit		
Vegetable		
Fat		

Meal 3	Time:	How do you feel during?
Protein		
Fruit		
Vegetable		
Fat		

Snack	Time:	How do you feel after?
Protein		
Vegetable		

Day 28

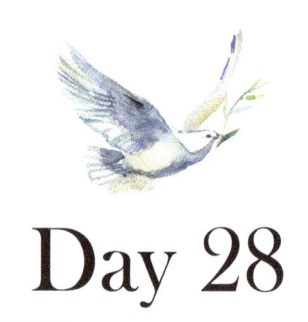

Date: _____

Exodus 15:26 (NIV)

He said, "If you listen carefully to the LORD your God and do what is right in his eyes, if you pay attention to his commands and keep all his decrees, I will not bring on you any of the diseases I brought on the Egyptians, for I am the LORD, who heals you."

GOD'S DESIRE FOR us is to be healthy and whole. He wants us to listen to Him. We should be spending time in the Word and in prayer to learn to hear Him. God speaks to us through His word, and sometimes in a still small voice during prayer. He also wants us to do what He views as right. The only way to know what is right in His eyes is to be in His Word daily.

When walking with God you will feel peace. We learn in Exodus that God will strive with us and go ahead of us. He will protect and fight for us.

Most emotions come and go. I find that when walking with God daily my predominant emotions are LOVE, JOY, and PEACE.

What is preventing these 3 emotions from being with you daily?

_____
_____
_____

What are you grateful for?

_____
_____
_____

Prayer Request

_____
_____
_____

Food Journal		Movement
Water _ _ _ _ _ _ _ _ _ _ _ _ _		**Rest Day**
		You can do Active Rest

Meal 1	Time:	
Protein		Walk at a slow pace.
Fruit		Low impact hiking
Vegetable		Low impact biking
Fat		

Meal 2	Time:	How do you feel before?
Protein		
Fruit		
Vegetable		
Fat		

Meal 3	Time:	How do you feel during?
Protein		
Fruit		
Vegetable		
Fat		

Snack	Time:	How do you feel after?
Protein		
Vegetable		

Day 29

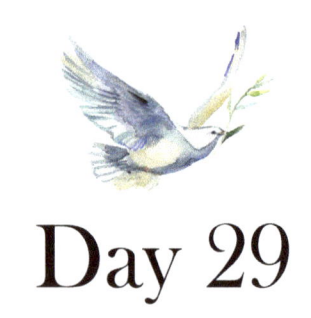

Date: _____

Isaiah 26:3 (NIV)
You will keep in perfect peace those whose minds are steadfast, because they trust in you.

WHY DO WE walk around in turmoil? Why do we worry?

In today's world we have so many things cluttering our minds like social media and the news. We spend too much time concerned about what others think of us. We worry about what others are doing. If we set our minds on the Word of the Lord and keep positive music and Godly things around us, He says we will have peace.

The things of the world do not bring love, joy or peace; but the Word of the Lord will calm and restore.

What are you filling your life with today? What can you replace in your life with God's love, joy, and peace?

_____
_____
_____

What are you grateful for?

_____
_____
_____

Prayer Request

_____
_____
_____

Food Journal	Movement
Water _ _ _ _ _ _ _ _ _ _ _ _	**Cardio** 30 minutes
	What Type:

Meal 1	Time:	How do you feel before?
Protein		
Fruit		
Vegetable		
Fat		

Meal 2	Time:	How do you feel during?
Protein		
Fruit		
Vegetable		
Fat		

Meal 3	Time:	How do you feel after?
Protein		
Fruit		
Vegetable		
Fat		

Snack	Time:
Protein	
Vegetable	

Day 30

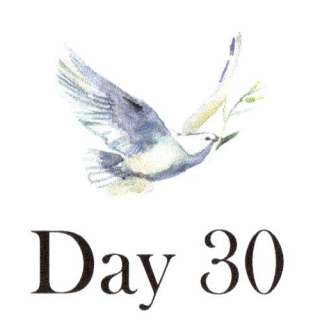

Date: _____

Psalms 145:14 (NIV)
The LORD upholds all who fall and lifts up all who are bowed down.

THE MORE TIME we spend each day in God's Word the more we begin to know what He wants, what He desires. When we fall or when the world is beating on us, God is there to hold us and help us through it. Helping us to not fall into temptation.

Stay close to Him and watch how He can lift you up in a storm.

What temptations do you seem to face each day? What are storms you are struggling with today? What will you do to prevent falling into temptation?

_____
_____
_____

What are you grateful for?

_____
_____
_____

Prayer Request

_____
_____
_____

Do you have any Prayer Requests that have been answered in the past 30 days?

_____
_____
_____

Food Journal		Movement
Water _ _ _ _ _ _ _ _ _ _ _ _		**Upper Body:** 3 sets of 12 each exercise
Meal 1	Time:	Bent over Rows
Protein		Bicep Curls Wide Grip Barbell
Fruit		Hammer Curls
Vegetable		Lat Pull Downs
Fat		Seated Rows

Meal 2	Time:	How do you feel before?
Protein		
Fruit		
Vegetable		
Fat		

Meal 3	Time:	How do you feel during?
Protein		
Fruit		
Vegetable		
Fat		

Snack	Time:	How do you feel after?
Protein		
Vegetable		

Day 31

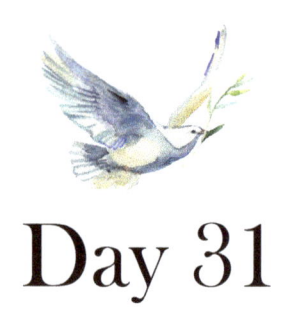

Date: _____

1 Corinthians 10:13 (NIV)
No temptation has overtaken you except what is common to mankind. And God is faithful; he will not let you be tempted beyond what you can bear. But when you are tempted, he will also provide a way out so that you can endure it.

Temptation aka Distraction

DISTRACTIONS CAN BE a form of temptation. You see satan does not want us to be on the path God wants us on. There will be things that will come up that God will allow to help you build faith in Him. God will always give you an escape route from temptation or distraction. You must be willing and ready to take the route He provides. It will always be better than taking the wrong turn.

Continue each day in the word and prayer to make sure you make the right decision and correct steps to prevent some of your own self-inflicted temptations.

How often do you make decisions without thinking about if this will be a distraction or a correct path?

_____
_____
_____

What are you grateful for?

_____
_____
_____

Prayer Request

_____
_____
_____

Food Journal			Movement
Water _ _ _ _ _ _ _ _ _ _ _			**HIIT**
Meal 1	Time:		Exercise 1:
Protein			Exercise 2:
			Exercise 3:
Fruit			Exercise 4:
Vegetable			Exercise 5:
Fat			

Meal 2	Time:	How do you feel before?
Protein		
Fruit		
Vegetable		
Fat		

Meal 3	Time:	How do you feel during?
Protein		
Fruit		
Vegetable		
Fat		

Snack	Time:	How do you feel after?
Protein		
Vegetable		

Day 32

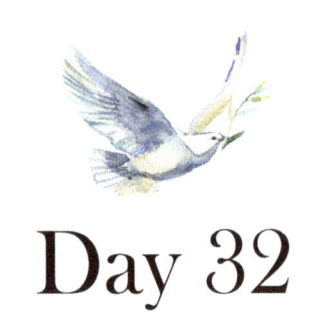

Date: _____

Galatians 5:22-23 (NIV)

22 But the fruit of the Spirit is love, joy, peace, forbearance, kindness, goodness, faithfulness, 23 gentleness and self-control. Against such things there is no law.

WHAT DO YOU spend most of the day thinking about? Are you focused on what others are thinking of you or how you feel about other people? Could you be drowning in past failures, worried to no end about bills, or wishing your work life was anything other than what it is?

Here is a thought, if you redirected your time on positive things how much fruit would you gain in your spirit? Know you are God's child! He created you and gave you an amazing personality and many talents. So don't waste time on things that are not of the Spirit.

This week, spend time on things of the Spirit. Where can you serve? What can you do to minimize self-inflicted actions? How can I better myself for God? Let the fruits flow through you.

Are you a good steward of God's time and money? _____

Do you gossip at home or work? _____

Do you give 100% of your accuracy at work? _____

Did God forgive your past failures? _____

Do you think about what others have? _____

What are you grateful for?

_____

_____

_____

Prayer Request

_____

_____

_____

Food Journal	**Movement**
Water _ _ _ _ _ _ _ _ _ _	**Cardio** 30 minutes
	What Type:

Meal 1	Time:	How do you feel before?
Protein		
Fruit		
Vegetable		
Fat		

Meal 2	Time:	How do you feel before?
Protein		
Fruit		
Vegetable		
Fat		

Meal 3	Time:	How do you feel during?
Protein		
Fruit		
Vegetable		
Fat		

Snack	Time:
Protein	
Vegetable	

Day 33

Date: _____

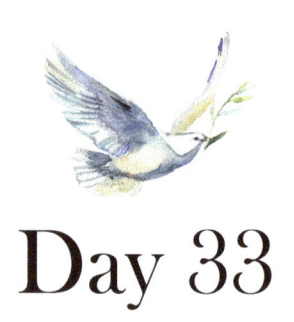

Proverbs 25:16 (NIV)

If you find honey, eat just enough— too much of it, and you will vomit.

LOOK AROUND YOU at the population of Americans in our world today. Nationally, 41.9% of adults are obese. Black adults had the highest level of adult obesity at 49.9%. Hispanic adults had an obesity rate of 45.6% and White adults had an obesity rate of 41.4%. These statistics are from September 27, 2022 and were obtained from the Trust for American Health. Not only do we as a nation overeat, but we overspend, and we collect "stuff" unnecessarily. We waste so much on things.

Today I will look at my life:

How do I eat? Do I overeat? Do I restrict for self-vanity?

_____
_____
_____

Do I spend wisely? _____
Do I use what I have to the fullest? _____
Do I use my time wisely? Where can I change my schedule? _____
Do I binge on social media, TV, or sleeping? _____

What are you grateful for?

_____
_____
_____

Prayer Request

_____
_____
_____

Food Journal		Movement	
Water _ _ _ _ _ _ _ _ _ _ _		**Lower Body:** 3 sets of 12 each exercise	
Meal 1	Time:	Exercise 1:	
Protein		Exercise 2:	
Fruit		Exercise 3:	
		Exercise 4:	
Vegetable		Exercise 5:	
Fat			

Meal 2	Time:	How do you feel before?
Protein		
Fruit		
Vegetable		
Fat		

Meal 3	Time:	How do you feel during?
Protein		
Fruit		
Vegetable		
Fat		

Snack	Time:	How do you feel after?
Protein		
Vegetable		

Day 34

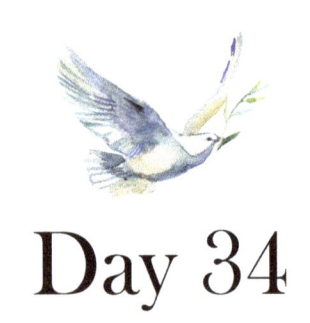

Date: _____

Exodus 23:1 (NIV)
"Do not spread false reports. Do not help a guilty person by being a malicious witness.

HOW MANY TIMES do we just simply *"state a fact"* about another saying: I'm not gossiping just *"stating a fact"*? Also, how many times do we just outright gossip?

This passage hit me hard when I read it. I felt that if what I was saying was true, it should be ok to tell it to others. I was wrong. God does not want us to gossip. If we are "stating facts" that cause harm to others we are tearing down and not building up. We should lift others. The old saying "if you can't say something nice, then don't say it at all" is truth.

Today only speak the truth in a way that lifts others when talking to friends and family.

Where can you improve in this area of your life?
_____

What are you grateful for?
_____
_____
_____

Prayer Request
_____
_____
_____

Food Journal		Movement	
Water _ _ _ _ _ _ _ _ _ _ _ _		**HIIT**	
Meal 1	Time:	Exercise 1:
Protein		Exercise 2:
		Exercise 3:
Fruit		Exercise 4:
Vegetable		Exercise 5:
Fat		

Meal 2	Time:	How do you feel before?
Protein		
Fruit		
Vegetable		
Fat		

Meal 3	Time:	How do you feel during?
Protein		
Fruit		
Vegetable		
Fat		

Snack	Time:	How do you feel after?
Protein		
Vegetable		

Day 35

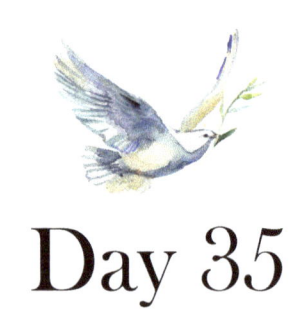

Date: _____

Proverbs 28:14 (NIV)

Blessed is the one who always trembles before God, but whoever hardens their heart falls into trouble.

AS WE WALK through life, we experience pain and sadness. People will hurt us and create wounds. If we do not take the pain of the world to the alter and lay them down, we will begin to get hard-hearted. Don't allow the evil of the world to harden your heart. Open yourself to God, lay the pain down and ask him to guard you as you walk through each day. Ask Him to move people and things that would harm you while setting the path that He would have you take to avoid evil. His path will always be the best for you.

Walk in the mercy and grace of God.

Are you holding in pain? Are you holding in resentments? What can you let go?

_____
_____
_____

What are you grateful for?

_____
_____
_____

Prayer Request

_____
_____
_____

Food Journal	Movement
Water _ _ _ _ _ _ _ _ _ _	**Rest Day**
	You can do Active Rest

Meal 1	Time:	
Protein		Walk at a slow pace.
Fruit		Low impact hiking
Vegetable		Low impact biking
Fat		

Meal 2	Time:	How do you feel before?
Protein		
Fruit		
Vegetable		
Fat		

Meal 3	Time:	How do you feel during?
Protein		
Fruit		
Vegetable		
Fat		

Snack	Time:	How do you feel after?
Protein		
Vegetable		

Day 36

Date: _____

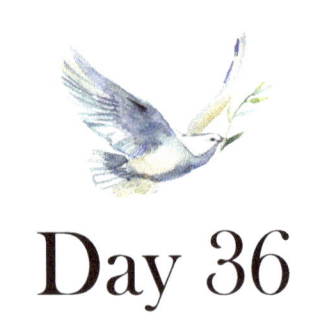

Ephesians 2:4-5 (NIV)

4 But because of his great love for us, God, who is rich in mercy 5 made us alive with Christ even when we were dead in transgressions—it is by grace you have been saved.

WHAT ARE YOU holding onto of which you need to let go? What have you not asked forgiveness for that is holding you back from being closer to God? God's mercy is ready to cleanse and heal you. Come alive today and allow God's mercy and grace to forgive and save you.

List the things you are holding on to. Then pray to let them go in Christ's name.

_____
_____
_____

What are you grateful for?

_____
_____
_____

Prayer Request

_____
_____
_____

Food Journal	Movement
Water __ __ __ __ __ __ __ __ __ __	**Cardio** 30 minutes
	What Type:

Meal 1	Time:	How do you feel before?
Protein		
Fruit		
Vegetable		
Fat		

Meal 2	Time:	How do you feel during?
Protein		
Fruit		
Vegetable		
Fat		

Meal 3	Time:	How do you feel after?
Protein		
Fruit		
Vegetable		
Fat		

Snack	Time:
Protein	
Vegetable	

Day 37

Date: _____

Romans 15:13 (NIV)

May the God of hope fill you with all joy and peace as you trust in him, so that you may overflow with hope by the power of the Holy Spirit.

WALKING IN THE Word each day is a new treasure. As we get closer to Him, joy and peace become more prevalent. We find situations less worrisome, and we get through them with more dignity.

I realized this during a dream. I watched myself and how I would have responded in the past. Then I sat back and realized this is not how I would respond today. I wanted to correct myself throughout the entire dream but could not reach the person I was watching. The pain I felt, the insecurities, and anger were all so much more. As I now align myself each day with God, I find I make better decisions. I feel more confident and have peace and joy beyond anything I have ever known.

Does that mean that I don't fall? No! I absolutely do! I just do not dwell on it like I did before. Do I get sad sometimes? Yes, but again I turn the thoughts to align with God's Word and overwhelming joy begins to fill me up.

Meditate on how you make decisions. Do you stop to align your decisions with God's Word? List some decisions you are currently making right now, and how they align with the word.

_____
_____
_____

What are you grateful for?

_____
_____
_____

Prayer Request

_____
_____
_____

Food Journal		Movement
Water _ _ _ _ _ _ _ _ _ _ _ _ _ _		**Upper Body:** 3 sets of 12 each exercise
Meal 1	Time:	Exercise 1: Exercise 2: Exercise 3: Exercise 4: Exercise 5:
Protein		
Fruit		
Vegetable		
Fat		

Meal 2	Time:	How do you feel before?
Protein		
Fruit		
Vegetable		
Fat		

Meal 3	Time:	How do you feel during?
Protein		
Fruit		
Vegetable		
Fat		

Snack	Time:	How do you feel after?
Protein		
Vegetable		

Day 38

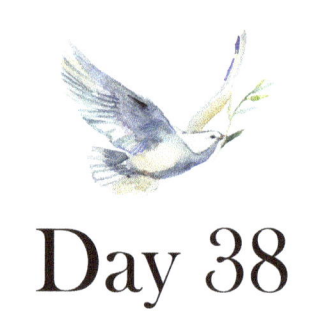

Date: _____

<u>**James 1:2-3 (NIV)**</u>
2 Consider it pure joy, my brothers and sisters, whenever you face trials of many kinds 3 because you know that the testing of your faith produces perseverance.

WE WILL FOREVER, for as long as we are on the earth, have trials and temptations. How we handle these times will bring joy or turmoil. The one thing you can count on is that when you are walking in the Word, satan is not going to like it. He will try to throw everything, including the kitchen sink at you.

Stand! Pray! Seek God's way! Look for the path that will bring Joy. Find the path that will lead you away from temptation and through the trials. Endure and find joy. Perseverance in faith will build strength.

What turmoil have you gone through recently? Look back and meditate on how you can change the next situation you encounter.

_____
_____
_____

What are you grateful for?

_____
_____
_____

Prayer Request

_____
_____
_____

Food Journal		**Movement**
Water _ _ _ _ _ _ _ _ _ _ _ _ _		**HIIT**
Meal 1	Time:	Exercise 1:
Protein		Exercise 2:
		Exercise 3:
Fruit		Exercise 4:
Vegetable		Exercise 5:
Fat		

Meal 2	Time:	How do you feel before?
Protein		
Fruit		
Vegetable		
Fat		

Meal 3	Time:	How do you feel during?
Protein		
Fruit		
Vegetable		
Fat		

Snack	Time:	How do you feel after?
Protein		
Vegetable		

Day 39

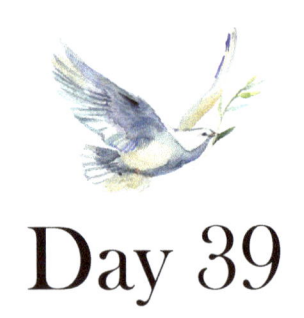

Date: _____

Philippians 4:4-6 (NIV)

Rejoice in the Lord always. I will say it again: Rejoice! Let your gentleness be evident to all. The Lord is nearby. Do not be anxious about anything, but in every situation, by prayer and petition, with thanksgiving, present your request to God.

REJOICE! KNOWING THAT God is always there. Do you struggle with anxiety? Do you struggle worrying? We don't need to. If we are walking in the light of the Lord, allowing Him to dictate our steps we can petition our request and God hears them. Not all our requests will be answered immediately or in the way we expect. Be open. Be willing to accept what God offers. It will be far better than we can imagine. If the answer is no, then it was not the path you needed to walk.

Are you walking in His light? Are you letting worldly views cloud your judgement and decisions? Is there something you need to lay down at the cross in order to ask for forgiveness?

_____
_____
_____

What are you grateful for?

_____
_____
_____

Prayer Request

_____
_____
_____

Food Journal	**Movement**
Water __ __ __ __ __ __ __ __ __ __	**Cardio** 30 minutes
	What Type:

Meal 1	Time:	How do you feel before?
Protein		
Fruit		
Vegetable		
Fat		

Meal 2	Time:	How do you feel during?
Protein		
Fruit		
Vegetable		
Fat		

Meal 3	Time:	How do you feel after?
Protein		
Fruit		
Vegetable		
Fat		

Snack	Time:	
Protein		
Vegetable		

Day 40

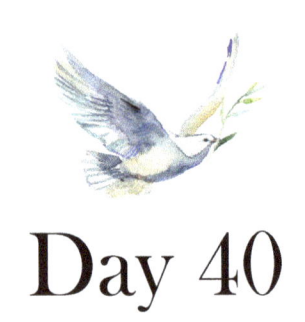

Date: _____

Psalms 16:7-11 (NIV)

"I will praise the Lord, who counsels me; even at night my heart instructs me. I keep my eyes always on the Lord. With Him at my right hand, I will not be shaken. Therefore, my heart is glad and my tongue rejoices; my body also will rest secure, because you will not abandon me to the realm of the dead, nor will you let your faithful one see decay. You make known to me the path of life; you will fill me with joy in your presence, with eternal pleasures at your right hand."

GOD TELLS US in this scripture why it's so important to keep seeking Him. He keeps us away from danger, sin, and corruption. Things we choose to do on our own out of His light will bring decay and turmoil. This is how we get depressed, anxious, and in trouble. When we choose to go the worldly route or do as we want to do, we never know what is going to happen. We lose the joy God brings us. Allow God daily to move you and move people in and out of your life.

What can you do today to begin to allow God to move you?

_____
_____
_____

What are you grateful for?

_____
_____
_____

Prayer Request

_____
_____
_____

Food Journal		**Movement**
Water _ _ _ _ _ _ _ _ _ _ _ _ _ _ _		**HIIT**
Meal 1	Time:	Exercise 1:
Protein		Exercise 2:
Fruit		Exercise 3:
	Exercise 4:
Vegetable		Exercise 5:
Fat		

Meal 2	Time:	How do you feel before?
Protein		
Fruit		
Vegetable		
Fat		

Meal 3	Time:	How do you feel during?
Protein		
Fruit		
Vegetable		
Fat		

Snack	Time:	How do you feel after?
Protein		
Vegetable		

Day 41

Date: _____

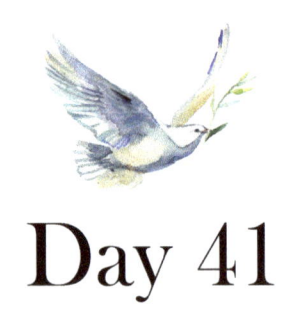

<u>**Luke 1:37 (NIV)**</u>
For no word from God will ever fail.

HERE WE READ God's word never fails. However, if we choose to not obey then the Word does not fail, we do. Before you take a step or speak, make sure you are not walking or speaking outside of the Word. In today's world we are tempted to have the last word. We are so busy we don't take time to listen or even think about how we should seek God's Word.

Today meditate on the word and slow yourself allowing the word to rise in you.

What does this passage say to you?

_____
_____
_____

What are you grateful for?

_____
_____
_____

Prayer Request

_____
_____
_____

Food Journal		**Movement**
Water _ _ _ _ _ _ _ _ _ _ _ _		Lower Body: 3 sets of 12 each exercise
Meal 1	Time:	Exercise 1: Exercise 2: Exercise 3: Exercise 4: Exercise 5:
Protein		
Fruit		
Vegetable		
Fat		

Meal 2	Time:	How do you feel before?
Protein		
Fruit		
Vegetable		
Fat		

Meal 3	Time:	How do you feel during?
Protein		
Fruit		
Vegetable		
Fat		

Snack	Time:	How do you feel after?
Protein		
Vegetable		

Day 42

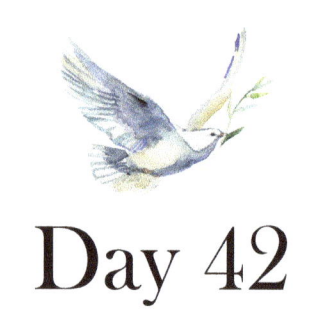

Date: _____

2 Corinthians 5:7-9 (NIV)
"For we live by faith, not by sight. We are confident, I say, and would prefer to be away from the body and at home with the Lord. So, we make it our goal to please him, whether we are at home in the body or away from it."

HERE THE BODY, I believe, is other people around you. The body of Christ. We all sin and fall short of the glory of God. So sometimes we don't want to be around others. We want to be safely hidden away in the presence of our Father God. We know if we are alone, it is easier to resist evil, be present, and please Him. However, we cannot stay hidden away. Make sure you reach for God's power and walk BOLDLY in the Spirit within you.

How often do you seclude yourself from others? Do you allow the trappings of the world to scare you away from going where God leads you? Do you take time to reach for the power of the Holy Spirit that dwells in you?

_____
_____
_____

What are you grateful for?

_____
_____
_____

Prayer Request

_____
_____
_____

Food Journal	Movement
Water _ _ _ _ _ _ _ _ _ _	**Rest Day**
	You can do Active Rest

Meal 1	Time:	
Protein		Walk at a slow pace.
Fruit		Low impact hiking
Vegetable		Low impact biking
Fat		

Meal 2	Time:	How do you feel before?
Protein		
Fruit		
Vegetable		
Fat		

Meal 3	Time:	How do you feel during?
Protein		
Fruit		
Vegetable		
Fat		

Snack	Time:	How do you feel after?
Protein		
Vegetable		

Day 43

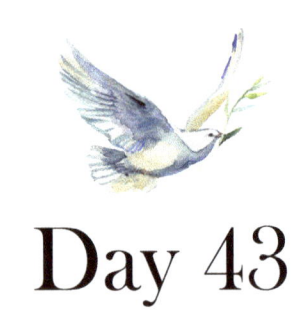

Date: _____

Matthew 21:22 (NIV)
If you believe, you will receive whatever you ask for in prayer."

THIS VERSE IS so true; however, keep it in context. We should be asking for things while using the Word as our guide. God understands the desires of our heart, but those desires should line up with His Word.

Do you want a car? That's ok, but don't be greedy? Do you need a high-end car if you've not been a good steward of your money? Yes, transportation is necessary, but could you easily use public transportation while saving, and being a good steward. Seek first what is good and pure, then ask for what is necessary.

Are you living your life lined up with the word? What are you asking of God? Is the request selfish? Are these requests honorable?

___

What are you grateful for?

___

Prayer Request

Food Journal		Movement
Water _ _ _ _ _ _ _ _ _ _ _ _		**Cardio** 30 minutes
		What Type:

Meal 1	Time:	How do you feel before?
Protein		
Fruit		
Vegetable		
Fat		

Meal 2	Time:	How do you feel during?
Protein		
Fruit		
Vegetable		
Fat		

Meal 3	Time:	How do you feel after?
Protein		
Fruit		
Vegetable		
Fat		

Snack	Time:
Protein	
Vegetable	

A DAILY WALK IN THE TEMPLE

Day 44

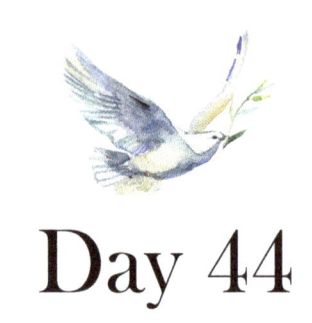

Date: _____

Romans 10:17 (NIV)

Consequently, faith comes from hearing the message, and the message is heard through the word about Christ.

SO, HOW DO you walk in faith. The first step is to read more and more of the Word. You need to learn, memorize, and hide the Word of God in your heart, mind, and soul. This way you will hear the Word and be able to live in faith. The word spells life out for us. We must walk in faith that the Word will play out in our lives.

How often do you spend memorizing and or reading the word of God?

_____
_____
_____

What are you grateful for?

_____
_____
_____

Prayer Request

_____
_____
_____

Food Journal		**Movement**
Water _ _ _ _ _ _ _ _ _ _ _ _		**HIIT**
Meal 1	Time:	Exercise 1:
Protein		Exercise 2:
Fruit		Exercise 3:
Vegetable		Exercise 4:
Fat		Exercise 5:

Meal 2	Time:	How do you feel before?
Protein		
Fruit		
Vegetable		
Fat		

Meal 3	Time:	How do you feel during?
Protein		
Fruit		
Vegetable		
Fat		

Snack	Time:	How do you feel after?
Protein		
Vegetable		

Day 45

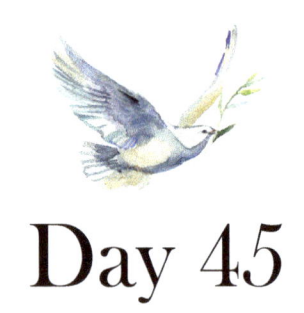

Date: _____

<u>Hebrews 11:6 (NIV)</u>
**And without faith it is impossible to please God,
because anyone who comes to him must believe that he exists and
that he rewards those who earnestly seek him.**

WE HAVE FAITH! We believe there is a God that loves us, and He sent His son Jesus as the ultimate sacrifice for our sin. We also believe that Jesus ascended into heaven and sent the Holy Spirit to reside in those who choose to believe and walk in the faith that the Word of God does not go void!

We find life's decisions become easier when we seek and spend time with Him daily. We have less stress because drama is at an all-time low. I am not saying we live happily ever after. We still are in the world. People want to watch us fail. That is sinful nature. People want to feel better about themselves, so they will start drama. If we are walking the right path God will have our back. Your reputation will go before you. People that walk in faith humble themselves. Become less of the world. Less of me and more of God equals a humble upright person.

Where do you fall short? Some people struggle with gossip, others with greed, some with stealing. What can God help you with today if you begin to boldly seek him? The sins of the world will become less and less in your life. Yes, we are human, we will fall. But your failures will not be as big as they used to be.

Meditate and write what comes to your mind after reading this devotion.

_____
_____
_____

What are you grateful for?

_____
_____
_____

Prayer Request

_____
_____
_____

Food Journal		Movement
Water _ _ _ _ _ _ _ _ _ _ _		**Upper Body:** 3 sets of 12 each exercise
Meal 1	Time:	Exercise 1: Exercise 2: Exercise 3: Exercise 4: Exercise 5:
Protein		
Fruit		
Vegetable		
Fat		

Meal 2	Time:	How do you feel before?
Protein		
Fruit		
Vegetable		
Fat		

Meal 3	Time:	How do you feel during?
Protein		
Fruit		
Vegetable		
Fat		

Snack	Time:	How do you feel after?
Protein		
Vegetable		

Day 46

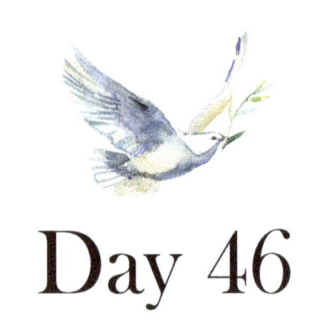

Date: _____

Psalms 118:24 (NIV)
The LORD has done it this very day; let us rejoice toDay and be glad.

WE WAKE UP on the wrong side of the bed some mornings. Fortunately for us God never does. The wonderful thing about God is He is always there to help set our mind right.

If we rejoice when we wake, we will not have room for negative emotions at that moment. Rejoice in the Lord until you feel the Spirit begin to rise and then go about your day.

What do you have today that's holding you back from rejoicing? Nothing should hold you back. God is ready to meet you where you are. Just let it out!!!!

Start here.

What are you grateful for?

_____
_____
_____

Prayer Request

_____
_____
_____

Food Journal	**Movement**
Water _ _ _ _ _ _ _ _ _ _ _	**Cardio** 30 minutes
	What Type:

Meal 1	Time:	How do you feel before?
Protein		
Fruit		
Vegetable		
Fat		

Meal 2	Time:	How do you feel during?
Protein		
Fruit		
Vegetable		
Fat		

Meal 3	Time:	How do you feel after?
Protein		
Fruit		
Vegetable		
Fat		

Snack	Time:	
Protein		
Vegetable		

Day 47

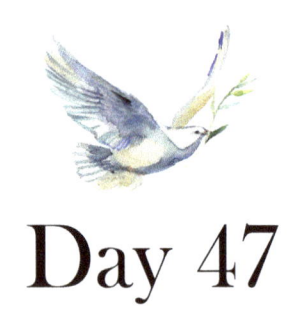

Date: _____

Revelation 17:14 (NIV)

They will wage war against the Lamb, but the Lamb will triumph over them because he is Lord of lords and King of kings—and with him will be his called, chosen and faithful followers."

DURING OUR LIVES we fight many temptations and battles with people around us and with things of the world. We fight doubts, fears, and anger. We forget to lean into God and remember that through Christ we can overcome all these obstacles. The Lamb goes before us paving the way. Seek Him to help guide you. You will win more battles and begin to triumph over temptation more often.

What can you do each day to slow down and seek God more?

_____
_____
_____

What are you grateful for?

_____
_____
_____

Prayer Request

_____
_____
_____

Food Journal		Movement
Water _ _ _ _ _ _ _ _ _ _ _ _		**HIIT**
Meal 1	Time:	Exercise 1:
Protein		Exercise 2:
Fruit		Exercise 3:
Vegetable		Exercise 4:
		Exercise 5:
Fat		

Meal 2	Time:	How do you feel before?
Protein		
Fruit		
Vegetable		
Fat		

Meal 3	Time:	How do you feel during?
Protein		
Fruit		
Vegetable		
Fat		

Snack	Time:	How do you feel after?
Protein		
Vegetable		

Day 48

Date: _____

John 16:33 (NIV)
"I have told you these things, so that in me you may have peace. In this world you will have trouble. But take heart! I have overcome the world."

THIS WORLD WAS perfect in the beginning. Then humans decided to sin. Now, we live in sin. Thankfully, God still gives us a way to be at peace. We have a choice to live in peace or live in strife. I can tell you that when I take matters into my own hands, life is much harder. When I wait and meditate on God, I am given a better way and have a peace that passes all understanding.

Today wait and reflect on how to handle situations. Then respond with God in you. Are you in a situation now that you need to seek God?

_____
_____
_____

What are you grateful for?

_____
_____
_____

Prayer Request

_____
_____
_____

Food Journal		**Movement**
Water _ _ _ _ _ _ _ _ _ _ _ _		**Lower Body:** 3 sets of 12 each exercise
Meal 1	Time:	Exercise 1:
Protein		Exercise 2:
		Exercise 3:
Fruit		Exercise 4:
Vegetable		Exercise 5:
Fat		

Meal 2	Time:	How do you feel before?
Protein		
Fruit		
Vegetable		
Fat		

Meal 3	Time:	How do you feel during?
Protein		
Fruit		
Vegetable		
Fat		

Snack	Time:	How do you feel after?
Protein		
Vegetable		

Day 49

Date: _____

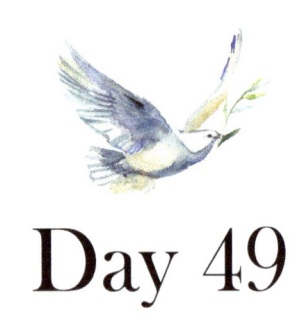

Matthew 6:33 (NIV)
But seek first his kingdom and his righteousness, and all these things will be given to you as well.

Who are you?
What do you want to accomplish?
Have you set goals?
What is the foundation in your life that keeps you safe, full of joy, and pushes you to be the best you can be?

WE GET SO busy in our daily lives that we forget to take time to remember the answers to the questions above. We also forget to thank and seek our Father who is our foundation. So, when we get down or in a fit of chaos, we should begin to seek Him.

How much stronger would you be against temptation and the world if you sought God?

_____

What are you grateful for?

_____
_____
_____

Prayer Request

_____
_____
_____

Food Journal		Movement
Water _ _ _ _ _ _ _ _ _ _ _ _ _		**Rest Day**
		You can do Active Rest

Meal 1	Time:	
Protein		Walk at a slow pace.
Fruit		Low impact hiking
Vegetable		Low impact biking
Fat		

Meal 2	Time:	How do you feel before?
Protein		
Fruit		
Vegetable		
Fat		

Meal 3	Time:	How do you feel during?
Protein		
Fruit		
Vegetable		
Fat		

Snack	Time:	How do you feel after?
Protein		
Vegetable		

Day 50

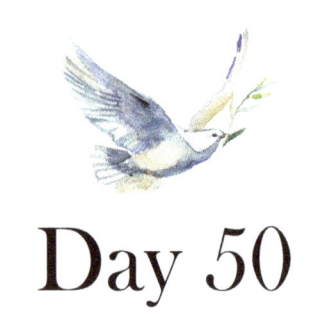

Date: _____

3 John 1:2 (NIV)

Dear friend, I pray that you may enjoy good health and that all may go well with you, even as your soul is getting along well.

WE ARE TOLD in several places in the Bible we should keep our bodies healthy. Here in the third chapter of John not only does he want our soul to be strong, but He also wants our body to be healthy, as well.

We cannot be prosperous in health if we are not a good steward of our body. Moving and eating clean is the way to be a good steward of your body.

How can you personally be a better steward of your body each day?

_____
_____
_____

What are you grateful for?

_____
_____
_____

Prayer Request

_____
_____
_____

Food Journal	Movement
Water __ __ __ __ __ __ __ __ __ __	**Cardio** 30 minutes
	What Type:

Meal 1	Time:	How do you feel before?
Protein		
Fruit		
Vegetable		
Fat		

Meal 2	Time:	How do you feel during?
Protein		
Fruit		
Vegetable		
Fat		

Meal 3	Time:	How do you feel after?
Protein		
Fruit		
Vegetable		
Fat		

Snack	Time:
Protein	
Vegetable	

Day 51

Date: _____

Psalms 16:1-2 (NIV)

Keep me safe, my God, for in you I take refuge. I say to the Lord, "You are my Lord; apart from you, I have no good thing."

DAVID KNEW HE could not make good decisions without the Lord. He was weak when he did not take refuge in God. He knew if he went before the Lord, confessed his sins, and made sacrifices, he would be forgiven. God loved David even though he sinned. God also loves all of us. Today, we are so blessed that Jesus made the ultimate sacrifice for us. Jesus' sacrifice made a way where we can go before the Lord and seek forgiveness for our sins. David tells us to take refuge in God. He will keep you safe. He will help you find the door to get away from the temptation. All you have to do is to take refuge.

What does taking refuge look like to you?

_____
_____
_____
_____

What are you grateful for?

_____
_____
_____

Prayer Request

_____
_____
_____

Food Journal		Movement
Water _ _ _ _ _ _ _ _ _ _ _ _		**HIIT**
Meal 1	Time:	Exercise 1:
Protein		Exercise 2:
		Exercise 3:
Fruit		Exercise 4:
Vegetable		Exercise 5:
Fat		

Meal 2	Time:	How do you feel before?
Protein		
Fruit		
Vegetable		
Fat		

Meal 3	Time:	How do you feel during?
Protein		
Fruit		
Vegetable		
Fat		

Snack	Time:	How do you feel after?
Protein		
Vegetable		

Day 52

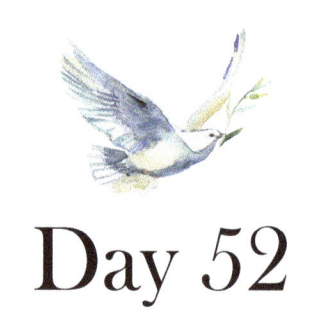

Date: _____

John 16:24 (NIV)
Until now you have not asked for anything in my name. Ask and you will receive, and your joy will be complete.

JESUS WAS SPEAKING to the disciples here. They have had Jesus by their side up to this point. They had faith in Jesus from being close to Him, being taught by Him, and watching the miracles He performed. Here Jesus is telling the disciples what is about to happen to Him, and how they will not be able to just walk and watch. They will have to walk in a different type of faith and ask for what they need. We, in the same way, must seek God each day and ask Him to guide our steps. We ask God to help us prevail over temptation. He promises us that He will bring us joy and help us if we just ask. Remember that some things take time. We may have to walk a while in faith. We learn as we stand and are patient.

What are you waiting for today? What do you feel you can do to help you stand in faith?

_____
_____
_____
_____

What are you grateful for?

_____
_____
_____

Prayer Request

_____
_____
_____

Food Journal		Movement
Water _ _ _ _ _ _ _ _ _ _ _ _ _ _		**Upper Body:** 3 sets of 12 each exercise
Meal 1	Time:	Exercise 1: Exercise 2: Exercise 3: Exercise 4: Exercise 5:
Protein		
Fruit		
Vegetable		
Fat		

Meal 2	Time:	How do you feel before?
Protein		
Fruit		
Vegetable		
Fat		

Meal 3	Time:	How do you feel during?
Protein		
Fruit		
Vegetable		
Fat		

Snack	Time:	How do you feel after?
Protein		
Vegetable		

Day 53

Date: _____

Romans 14:17-18 (NIV)

17 For the kingdom of God is not a matter of eating and drinking, but of righteousness, peace and joy in the Holy Spirit, 18 because anyone who serves Christ in this way is pleasing to God and receives human approval.

NOW, DO NOT take this verse and tell me you can eat and drink whatever you wish. I do not believe God was speaking to us about that. Here he is telling us that if we walk according to the Word and serve God, we will be pleasing to Him. During this time of life there were no processed foods, chemicals sprayed on foods, or fast food. I believe if you are serving God and being righteous, you will be less likely to be glutenous and damage your body. Many of us eat and overeat because we are depressed or bored. We also may starve ourselves because of the same reasons. What I believe God is telling us is that if we serve Him and truly strive to be righteous, our bodies will follow suit. We will not want to eat or starve ourselves because we will be at peace and have a joy that passes all understanding. We will be occupied with walking out his purpose.

Today meditate on how you can serve God, and what you can do to be righteous in His sight.

_____
_____
_____

What are you grateful for?

_____
_____
_____

Prayer Request

_____
_____
_____

Food Journal	**Movement**
Water _ _ _ _ _ _ _ _ _ _ _ _	**Cardio** 30 minutes
	What Type:

Meal 1	Time:	How do you feel before?
Protein		
Fruit		
Vegetable		
Fat		

Meal 2	Time:	How do you feel during?
Protein		
Fruit		
Vegetable		
Fat		

Meal 3	Time:	How do you feel after?
Protein		
Fruit		
Vegetable		
Fat		

Snack	Time:
Protein	
Vegetable	

Day 54

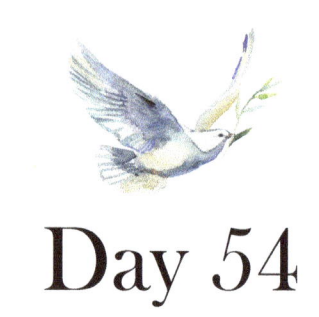

Date: _____

1 Peter 1:8 (NIV)

8 Though you have not seen him, you love him; and even though you do not see him now, you believe in him and are filled with an inexpressible and glorious joy, 9 for you are receiving the end result of your faith, the salvation of your souls.

EACH DAY, AS you wake and begin your journey with prayer and reading the Word, you will find your mind is opened to a new way of living. As you grow in your relationship with God you will experience less guilt, less shame, and less anxiety. You will begin to have more positive thoughts. You will not allow yourself to dwell on the evil of the world because you start to see the face of Jesus throughout your day. You will begin to make better choices. You will choose not to talk poorly of others. Temptation will be easier to handle because you seek Him first.

What are you seeing that is becoming easier the more you are walking in faith?

_____
_____
_____

What are you grateful for?

_____
_____
_____

Prayer Request

_____
_____
_____

Food Journal		Movement
Water __ __ __ __ __ __ __ __ __ __		**HIIT**
Meal 1	Time:	Exercise 1:
Protein		Exercise 2:
Fruit		Exercise 3:
Vegetable		Exercise 4:
		Exercise 5:
Fat		

Meal 2	Time:	How do you feel before?
Protein		
Fruit		
Vegetable		
Fat		

Meal 3	Time:	How do you feel during?
Protein		
Fruit		
Vegetable		
Fat		

Snack	Time:	How do you feel after?
Protein		
Vegetable		

Day 55

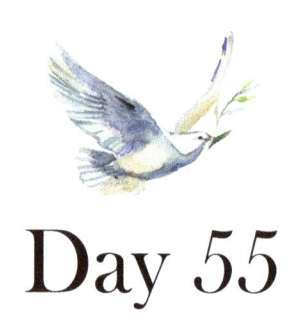

Date: _____

Nehemiah 8:10 (NIV)

Nehemiah said, "Go and enjoy choice food and sweet drinks, and send some to those who have nothing prepared. This Day is holy to our Lord. Do not grieve, for the joy of the LORD is your strength."

THROUGHOUT HISTORY FOOD and drinks have been for celebration. We should celebrate while bringing the best of the best to the table. Thinking about the best of the best, would you say processed foods would be on the table? There are sweets and breads that were delicious during that time, and we can make better choices if we take the time to cook with clean foods. I believe celebrations should not occur on a weekly basis. Celebrating is for holidays, birthdays, anniversaries, and even funerals. We see these types of feasts throughout the Bible. However, you would not see this way of eating daily or weekly. Food was fuel and it was necessary to be able to move each day for chores and spreading the gospel. People did not "exercise" like we do today because the day-to-day movement was extreme. Movement then, consisting of fishing, farming, harvesting, walking to the well, drawing water, and hand washing laundry was very different than we see today. Now, we sit most of the day and eat poor food choices.

What can you do during the day to prevent eating poorly, and what can you do to move more?

_____
_____
_____

What are you grateful for?

_____
_____
_____

Prayer Request

_____
_____
_____

Food Journal		**Movement**
Water _ _ _ _ _ _ _ _ _ _ _ _		Lower Body: 3 sets of 12 each exercise
Meal 1	Time:	Exercise 1:
Protein		Exercise 2:
Fruit		Exercise 3:
Vegetable		Exercise 4:
Fat		Exercise 5:

Meal 2	Time:	How do you feel before?
Protein		
Fruit		
Vegetable		
Fat		

Meal 3	Time:	How do you feel during?
Protein		
Fruit		
Vegetable		
Fat		

Snack	Time:	How do you feel after?
Protein		
Vegetable		

Day 56

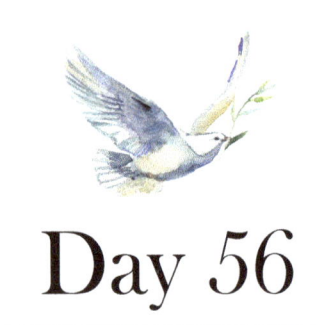

Date: _____

Zephaniah 3:17 (NIV)
**The LORD your God is with you, the Mighty Warrior who saves.
He will take great delight in you; in his love He will no longer rebuke you,
but will rejoice over you with singing."**

IF YOU BEGAN your journey 55 days ago, have been seeking God each day diligently, and are desiring to walk in the light of God, He sees your actions and is meeting you where you are. God is delighted in you and is ready to fight and win battles and wars for you. He is singing and rejoicing over you while He is with you. He will not rebuke your desires, and He longs to walk with you daily. Keep stepping towards Him and walking daily with Him. Journal the days and watch how you are growing. Watch how God is opening doors. Watch how things in your life continue to change for the better.

What are you still having difficulty letting go of?

_____

Do you still have questions that are not getting answered?

_____

What steps are you going to take to continue walking towards God even if the answers have not been presented?

_____

_____

What are you grateful for?

_____

_____

_____

Prayer Request

_____

_____

_____

Food Journal	Movement
Water _ _ _ _ _ _ _ _ _ _	**Rest Day**
	You can do Active Rest

Meal 1	Time:	
Protein		Walk at a slow pace.
Fruit		Low impact hiking
Vegetable		Low impact biking
Fat		

Meal 2	Time:	How do you feel before?
Protein		
Fruit		
Vegetable		
Fat		

Meal 3	Time:	How do you feel during?
Protein		
Fruit		
Vegetable		
Fat		

Snack	Time:	How do you feel after?
Protein		
Vegetable		

Day 57

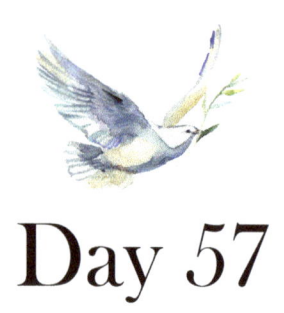

Date: _____

John 15:9-12 (NIV)

"As the Father has loved me, so have I loved you. Now remain in my love. If you keep my commands, you will remain in my love, just as I have kept my Father's command and remain in his love. I have told you this so that my joy may be in you and that your joy may be complete. My command is this: Love each other as I have loved you.

HERE IS A great love with the benefits of joy, peace, and forgiveness. I do believe that Jesus loves us even when we fall or fail to abide by his word. This does not mean we should give up trying to be better than the day before. Continue to love others like God loved His only child. Throughout Jesus' life God showed Jesus His love. God knew of every step Jesus took all the way to the cross where they were separated as Jesus took our sin upon Himself. Then, Jesus rose from the dead. He was redeemed and is sitting beside God, standing up for us when we ask forgiveness for our failures and sins.

Today how will you show others Jesus's love?

_____
_____
_____

What are you grateful for?

_____
_____
_____

Prayer Request

_____
_____
_____

Food Journal	**Movement**
Water _ _ _ _ _ _ _ _ _ _	**Cardio** 30 minutes
	What Type:

Meal 1	Time:	How do you feel before?
Protein		
Fruit		
Vegetable		
Fat		

Meal 2	Time:	How do you feel during?
Protein		
Fruit		
Vegetable		
Fat		

Meal 3	Time:	How do you feel after?
Protein		
Fruit		
Vegetable		
Fat		

Snack	Time:	
Protein		
Vegetable		

Day 58

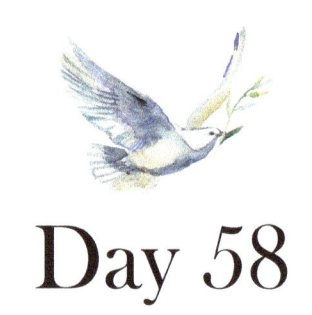

Date: _____

Psalms 51:12 (NIV)
Restore to me the joy of your salvation and grant me a willing spirit,
to sustain me.

REALIZE THAT GOD knows we are human. He knows when we sin. Please understand that this is not a game. He created us and gave us free will. He also wants to love us and walk with us. Ask Him each day to give you strength to sustain and to guide you so that you do not sin. Allow Him to move in you so you receive unspeakable joy.

Do you struggle somedays wondering why God created us knowing we would sin?
_____

Begin researching what the bible says regarding this and take notes at the back of the book. This is a good time to begin your journey researching the word.

What are you grateful for?
_____
_____
_____

Prayer Request
_____
_____
_____

Food Journal		Movement	
Water _ _ _ _ _ _ _ _ _ _ _		**HIIT**	
Meal 1	Time:	Exercise 1	
Protein		Exercise 2	
Fruit		Exercise 3	
Vegetable		Exercise 4	
Fat		Exercise 5	

Meal 2	Time:	How do you feel before?
Protein		
Fruit		
Vegetable		
Fat		

Meal 3	Time:	How do you feel during?
Protein		
Fruit		
Vegetable		
Fat		

Snack	Time:	How do you feel after?
Protein		
Vegetable		

Day 59

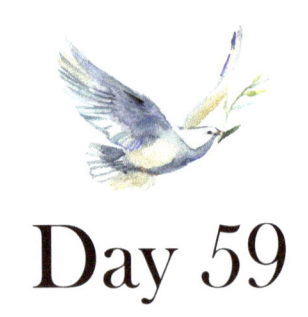

Date: _____

Psalms 28:1-2 (NIV)

To you, LORD, I call; you are my Rock, do not turn a deaf ear to me. For if you remain silent, I will be like those who go down to the pit. 2. Hear me cry for mercy as I call to you for help, as I lift up my hands toward your Most Holy Place.

ALL WE MUST do is repent and cry out to God. He is there. Don't get so far away from Him that you cannot feel His presence. The more we decide to do things on our own, or the more we sin, the further away from God we get. That can lead to feelings of guilt and shame. Today repent, cry out to God, and repent. Let Him be your rock. Lean into Him and call on Him daily. Ask that He not turn a deaf ear or remain silent.

Do you have times when you feel far away from God? Are you are too ashamed to go to Him? Lift your hands towards His Holy Place today and cry out. He is ready to meet you where you are to bring you back to peace.

What are you grateful for?

_____
_____
_____

Prayer Request

_____
_____
_____

Food Journal	Movement
Water _ _ _ _ _ _ _ _ _ _ _ _ _ _	**Upper Body:** 3 sets of 12 each exercise

Meal 1	Time:	
Protein		Exercise 1
Fruit		Exercise 2
Vegetable		Exercise 3
Fat		Exercise 4
		Exercise 5

Meal 2	Time:	How do you feel before?
Protein		
Fruit		
Vegetable		
Fat		

Meal 3	Time:	How do you feel during?
Protein		
Fruit		
Vegetable		
Fat		

Snack	Time:	How do you feel after?
Protein		
Vegetable		

Day 60

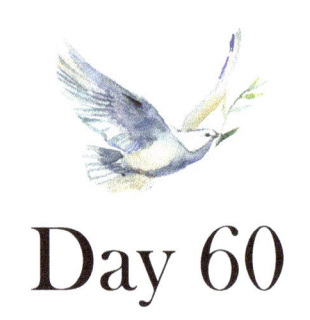

Date: _____

Psalms 28:7 (NIV)

The LORD is my strength and my shield; my heart trusts in him, and he helps me. My heart leaps for joy, and with my song I praise him.

What is your biggest weakness?

IS THERE A certain person, place, or thing that just pulls you away from God's presence? How can you begin to use God's strength to tear down this wall in your life. This weakness is not of God. Why do you keep yourself from joy and peace. Today, write it down. Then begin to seek God and watch a door begin to open. This is when you also pray for the strength to walk through the door. Allowing the person, place, or thing to be behind you and never to pick it up again.

Weakness brings guilt, shame, and loneliness. God brings joy, peace, and mercy.
What do you choose today?

What are you grateful for?

___

Prayer Request

Food Journal	**Movement**
Water __ __ __ __ __ __ __ __ __ __	**Cardio** 30 minutes
	What Type:

Meal 1	Time:	How do you feel before?
Protein		
Fruit		
Vegetable		
Fat		

Meal 2	Time:	How do you feel during?
Protein		
Fruit		
Vegetable		
Fat		

Meal 3	Time:	How do you feel after?
Protein		
Fruit		
Vegetable		
Fat		

Snack	Time:
Protein	
Vegetable	

Day 61

Date: _____

James 1:2-4 (NIV)
**Consider it pure joy, my brothers and sisters, whenever you face trials of many kinds, because you know that the testing of your faith produces perseverance.
Let perseverance finish its work so that you may be mature and complete,
not lacking anything.**

JUST LIKE AN Olympic athlete that trains for perfection to win the Gold Medal, we as Christians should train to be the best we can be as a human. The Olympian has trials; days he or she is extremely tired, a twist or turn that is difficult to master, or a time they struggle to beat. We also have trials and tests we must overcome without falling into temptation. These trials mold us. They teach us to seek God more quickly and to avoid falling into the traps of this world so we can endure to the end. Instead of a gold medal our prize is eternity with Jesus!

What are your most current temptations that you cannot seem to shake off?

_____
_____
_____

What are you grateful for?

_____
_____
_____

Prayer Request

_____
_____
_____

Food Journal			Movement	
Water _ _ _ _ _ _ _ _ _ _			**HIIT**	
Meal 1	Time:		Exercise 1:	
Protein			Exercise 2:	
			Exercise 3:	
Fruit			Exercise 4:	
Vegetable			Exercise 5:	
Fat				

Meal 2	Time:	How do you feel before?
Protein		
Fruit		
Vegetable		
Fat		

Meal 3	Time:	How do you feel during?
Protein		
Fruit		
Vegetable		
Fat		

Snack	Time:	How do you feel after?
Protein		
Vegetable		

A DAILY WALK IN THE TEMPLE ~ 123

Day 62

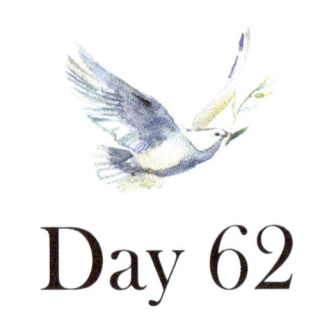

Date: _____

Hebrews 12:1-3 (NIV)

Therefore, since we are surrounded by such a great cloud of witnesses, let us throw off everything that hinders and the sin that so easily entangles. And let us run with perseverance the race marked out for us. Fixing our eyes on Jesus, the pioneer and perfecter of faith. For the joy set before Him He endured the cross, scorning its shame, and sat down at the right hand of the throne of God. Consider Him who endured such opposition from sinners, so that you will not grow weary and lose heart.

YES, WE ARE being watched each day by people around us. It often times seems like people would prefer to see someone fail rather than succeed. Social media has made this easier to watch and will at times glorify failure. What are you showing the people that are watching you? Do you start or engage in gossip? Do you follow all the trends to make sure no one sees you as different? Should you instead turn your back on the ways of the world and follow the one that hung on the cross? Should you follow the one that made the ultimate stand against the world. He endured so much so that we could have an easier way to walk and be found righteous.

Surround yourself with people that want you to succeed, people that seek God and not the world. Turn yourself away from the trappings of this world and be ready to show them Jesus. Even though some want you to fail, you still need to show love.

What are you grateful for?

_____
_____
_____

Prayer Request

_____
_____
_____

Food Journal	Movement
Water __ __ __ __ __ __ __ __ __ __ __	**Lower Body:** 3 sets of 12 each exercise

Meal 1	Time:	
Protein		Exercise 1
Fruit		Exercise 2
Vegetable		Exercise 3
Fat		Exercise 4
		Exercise 5

Meal 2	Time:	How do you feel before?
Protein		
Fruit		
Vegetable		
Fat		

Meal 3	Time:	How do you feel during?
Protein		
Fruit		
Vegetable		
Fat		

Snack	Time:	How do you feel after?
Protein		
Vegetable		

Day 63

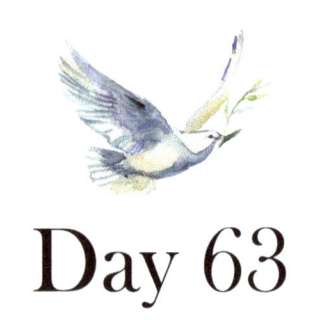

Date: _____

Proverbs 17:22 (NIV)
A cheerful heart is good medicine, but a crushed spirit dries up the bones.

WE LOVE TO be told how good we are doing or get a promotion at work. However, when we get reprimanded, we do not feel joyful. We should think about and recognize how we treat others. Do we lift up the people we are around, or do we bring them down? Do we cheer on our friends even if he or she may be going for the same position, or do we backstab them to make ourselves look better. God shows us here it is better to be cheerful and giving rather than backstabbing and hurtful.

Really look at yourself right now. How do you typically treat others? Where could you change?

What are you grateful for?

_____
_____
_____

Prayer Request

_____
_____
_____

Food Journal		**Movement**
Water _ _ _ _ _ _ _ _ _ _		**Rest Day**
		You can do Active Rest

Meal 1	Time:	
Protein		Walk at a slow pace.
Fruit		Low impact hiking
Vegetable		Low impact biking
Fat		

Meal 2	Time:	How do you feel before?
Protein		
Fruit		
Vegetable		
Fat		

Meal 3	Time:	How do you feel during?
Protein		
Fruit		
Vegetable		
Fat		

Snack	Time:	How do you feel after?
Protein		
Vegetable		

Day 64

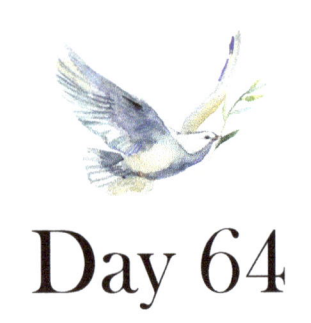

Date: _____

Proverbs 17:23-24 (NIV)

The wicked accept bribes in secret to pervert the course of justice. A discerning person keeps wisdom in view, but a fool's eyes wander to the ends of the earth.

THIS IS A great eye opener! How often do we see the wicked perverting and twisting things to get what they want. They make others seem less than and cause chaos. Do you want to pervert and twist or be wise? Do you want to bring peace and joy or chaos and destruction. Separate yourself from those accepting bribes or spreading gossip. If you are the one gossiping and harming others to feel better about yourself, take a step back and analyze your heart. Do you have past trauma you continue to ignore or don't fully understand? Do you feel neglected somewhere in your life? Take this to God and ask what needs to happen for restoration to occur. Ask God to take away the person that is in your life causing the chaos.

Write your thoughts:

_____
_____
_____

What are you grateful for?

_____
_____
_____

Prayer Request

_____
_____
_____

Food Journal	**Movement**
Water __ __ __ __ __ __ __ __ __ __	**Cardio** 30 minutes
	What Type:

Meal 1	Time:	How do you feel before?
Protein		
Fruit		
Vegetable		
Fat		

Meal 2	Time:	How do you feel during?
Protein		
Fruit		
Vegetable		
Fat		

Meal 3	Time:	How do you feel after?
Protein		
Fruit		
Vegetable		
Fat		

Snack	Time:
Protein	
Vegetable	

Day 65

Date: _____

Proverbs 10:28-29 (NIV)
The prospect of the righteous is joy, but the hopes of the wicked come to nothing. The way of the Lord is a refuge for the blameless, but it is the ruin of those who do evil.

STAY ON GOD'S path of light. It is a narrow path for certain. But His path is joyful. When we stray, we find nothing but ruin. I have found that when I decide to do things my way I destroy things in my life. It at times damages my family and friends. Not only do I hurt them, but I also lose their trust. How is this joyful? How is this peaceful? It is not. I do find that once I opened my eyes and the shackles were lifted, Jesus was there to forgive me. Jesus brought my joy back. Yes, I had consequences for sure. I had to tell the truth and ask for forgiveness not only from Jesus, but from my family and friends as well. I had to rebuild trust. Jesus does not just wipe the past away. He is there to help guide you and prepare the hearts of those you hurt. I am blessed to find joy and peace again. I pray each day that I do not allow myself to follow the worldly path again.

Notes:
_____
_____
_____

What are you grateful for?
_____
_____
_____

Prayer Request
_____
_____
_____

Food Journal		Movement
Water _ _ _ _ _ _ _ _ _ _		**HIIT**
Meal 1	Time:	Exercise 1:
Protein		Exercise 2:
Fruit		Exercise 3:
Vegetable		Exercise 4:
		Exercise 5:
Fat		

Meal 2	Time:	How do you feel before?
Protein		
Fruit		
Vegetable		
Fat		

Meal 3	Time:	How do you feel during?
Protein		
Fruit		
Vegetable		
Fat		

Snack	Time:	How do you feel after?
Protein		
Vegetable		

Day 66

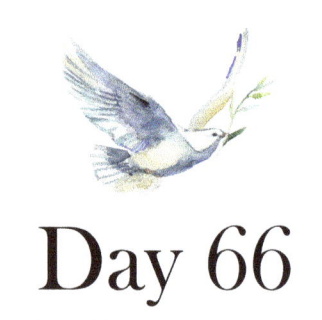

Date: _____

Proverbs 23:1-2 (NIV)
**When you sit to dine with a ruler, note well what is before you,
and put a knife to your throat if you are given to gluttony.**

GOD KNOWS WE can overeat and be gluttonous. God knows how you are created, and how overeating effects the human body. When you are celebrating, eat things you typically do not eat and enjoy them, but do not be gluttonous eating until you cannot move. Yes, celebrate, eat, and then let the food settle. If you feel you can eat a little more that is fine. It is not good for your body to consume so much food until you hurt. Your body is not created to be overfilled. Be aware of your body and your body's limits.

Do you take time to know how your body responds to foods you typically do not eat? By day 66 you have reduced processed foods greatly or have eliminated them all together. By now there is most likely some type of celebration about to occur. During this time eat slowly, feel how your body responds. Does the sugar make you feel heavy? Do you bloat? Begin to realize when you are full. You can always have one more meal of leftovers and then be done. Get all the treats or foods you do not need out of the house.

What are you grateful for?

_____
_____
_____

Prayer Request

_____
_____
_____

Food Journal	Movement
Water __ __ __ __ __ __ __ __ __ __ __ __	**Upper Body:** 3 sets of 12 each exercise

Meal 1	Time:	
Protein		Exercise 1
Fruit		Exercise 2
Vegetable		Exercise 3
Fat		Exercise 4
		Exercise 5

Meal 2	Time:	How do you feel before?
Protein		
Fruit		
Vegetable		
Fat		

Meal 3	Time:	How do you feel during?
Protein		
Fruit		
Vegetable		
Fat		

Snack	Time:	How do you feel after?
Protein		
Vegetable		

Day 67

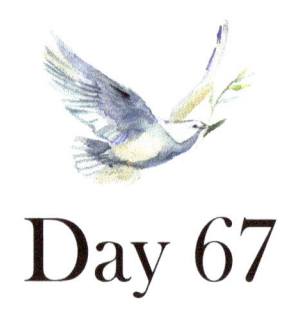

Date: _____

1 Peter 5:6-7 (NIV)

Humble yourselves, therefore, under God's mighty hand, that he may lift you up in due time. Cast all your anxiety on Him because He cares for you.

WE HAVE SO many things going on at one time it is crazy. What we need to do is let some of the frills go and humble ourselves. Let go of the bells and whistles we do not need. There are so many advertisements for food, jewelry, houses, and just about anything you can imagine. Do we cut it all off and spend time with God and realize that we are overloading ourselves with things of this world? Do you realize how much stress trying to keep up with the world's trappings puts on your mind and body? We end up spending more money than we make, which causes us to work more than we should. God can show you how life can be free of this stress if you just stop and be still. Seek what He would have you do with your time and money.

Today humble yourself and really think what you could let go that could bring you peace.

_____
_____
_____

What are you grateful for?

_____
_____
_____

Prayer Request

_____
_____
_____

Food Journal	Movement
Water _ _ _ _ _ _ _ _ _ _ _ _	**Cardio** 30 minutes
	What Type:

Meal 1	Time:	How do you feel before?
Protein		
Fruit		
Vegetable		
Fat		

Meal 2	Time:	How do you feel during?
Protein		
Fruit		
Vegetable		
Fat		

Meal 3	Time:	How do you feel after?
Protein		
Fruit		
Vegetable		
Fat		

Snack	Time:
Protein	
Vegetable	

Day 68

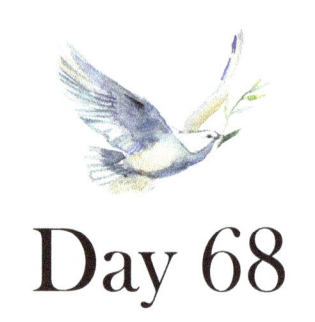

Date: _____

1 Peter 5:8-11 (NIV)

Be alert and sober of mind. Your enemy, the devil, prowls around like a roaring lion looking for someone to devour. Resist him, standing firm in the faith, because you know that the family of believers throughout the world is undergoing the same kind of sufferings. And the God of all grace, who called you to his eternal glory in Christ, after you have suffered a little while, will himself restore you and make you strong, firm and steadfast. To him be the power for ever and ever. Amen.

WE NEED TO understand that to be sober is not just about alcohol. It is anything you overindulge in and takes you away from time with God. It can be anything that draws you away from your purpose or path God has for you. When we take our focus off God's purpose and onto worldly things the enemy has a crack in the door he will use to gain entry. The enemy knows your thoughts and desires as well, he has his minions following you, lying to you, and watching you. These minions are ready to pounce and destroy what peace and joy you have. Be aware of the people and places you allow yourself to be around or enter. Be mindful of what you listen to as well. Stay focused and in prayer. Talk to God in good times and difficult times. The more you call on Him the closer you are to Him. Leave the doors shut to the enemy.

What are you allowing yourself to overindulge in that could be keeping you away from the purpose God has for you?

_____
_____
_____

What are you grateful for?

_____
_____
_____

Prayer Request

_____
_____
_____

Food Journal		**Movement**
Water _ _ _ _ _ _ _ _ _ _		**HIIT**
Meal 1	Time:	Exercise 1:
Protein		Exercise 2:
		Exercise 3:
Fruit		Exercise 4:
Vegetable		Exercise 5:
Fat		

Meal 2	Time:	How do you feel before?
Protein		
Fruit		
Vegetable		
Fat		

Meal 3	Time:	How do you feel during?
Protein		
Fruit		
Vegetable		
Fat		

Snack	Time:	How do you feel after?
Protein		
Vegetable		

Day 69

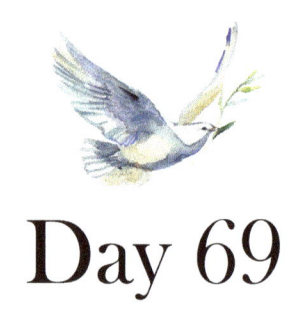

Date: _____

John 14:27 (NIV)

Peace, I leave with you; my peace I give you. I do not give to you as the world gives.
Do not let your hearts be troubled and do not be afraid.

OUR GOD TRULY wants us to live in peace. We are told this from the Old Testament through the New Testament. Here he explains that the peace he has for us is far better than that of the world. We can be of the world and have instant gratification depleting the peace in ourselves because we are always trying to keep up or get ahead. Or, we can choose not to overindulge on the worldly things and seek God while living in peace daily. Staying in prayer, reading the Word, and seeking God's peace is how we live out our purpose daily.

Notes from meditation:

_____
_____
_____

What are you grateful for?

_____
_____
_____

Prayer Request

_____
_____
_____

Food Journal		Movement
Water _ _ _ _ _ _ _ _ _ _		Lower Body: 3 sets of 12 each exercise
Meal 1	Time:	Exercise 1:
Protein		Exercise 2:
Fruit		Exercise 3:
Vegetable		Exercise 4:
		Exercise 5:
Fat		

Meal 2	Time:	How do you feel before?
Protein		
Fruit		
Vegetable		
Fat		

Meal 3	Time:	How do you feel during?
Protein		
Fruit		
Vegetable		
Fat		

Snack	Time:	How do you feel after?
Protein		
Vegetable		

Day 70

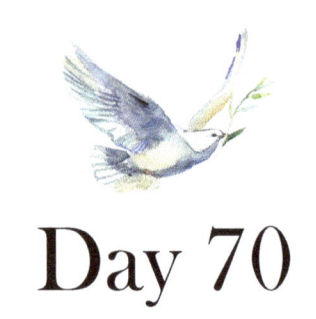

Date: _____

Matthew 6:34 (NIV)

Therefore, do not worry about tomorrow, for tomorrow will worry about itself. Each Day has enough trouble of its own.

GOD HAS A lot packed into this verse. How many times have you worried so much about a test or meeting that is a day away. Wasting time today that you could be walking in the light. Be prepared. Perhaps you have a task coming up. You should take steps to prepare and reduce stress. If you are giving 100 percent and are prepared your meeting should be of no stress to you. If you keep focus on what God has for you then you should be ready for what is about to come. God has prepared a way for you. Each day walk like there is not a tomorrow. Giving God all you have Today!

Notes from your meditation:

_____
_____
_____

What are you grateful for?

_____
_____
_____

Prayer Request

_____
_____
_____

Food Journal		Movement
Water _ _ _ _ _ _ _ _ _ _		**Rest Day**
		You can do Active Rest

Meal 1	Time:	
Protein		Walk at a slow pace.
Fruit		Low impact hiking
Vegetable		Low impact biking
Fat		

Meal 2	Time:	How do you feel before?
Protein		
Fruit		
Vegetable		
Fat		

Meal 3	Time:	How do you feel during?
Protein		
Fruit		
Vegetable		
Fat		

Snack	Time:	How do you feel after?
Protein		
Vegetable		

Day 71

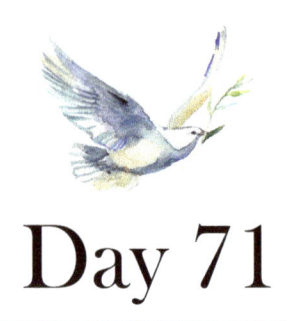

Date: _____

2 Timothy 1:7 (NIV)
**For the Spirit God gave us does not make us timid,
but gives us power, love, and self-discipline.**

WE HAVE THE POWER! You are a little over two months into a new lifestyle. Walking daily with God, eating cleaner, and moving more. You should feel amazing. You should be tapping into the power God is speaking of in this verse. When the drama of the world comes at you, reach within yourself and allow the Spirit of God to present! When you are weak, tired, or overwhelmed, stand and pray for the power to rise. Know the strength you have. Know you can tap into the power anytime you want. Stay close to God. Call on God all the time. Joyous times and difficult times are both times to call on God.

How are you responding to life today differently than you did 70 days ago?

_____
_____
_____

What are you grateful for?

_____
_____
_____

Prayer Request

_____
_____
_____

Food Journal	**Movement**
Water _ _ _ _ _ _ _ _ _ _ _ _	**Cardio** 30 minutes
	What Type:

Meal 1	Time:	How do you feel before?
Protein		
Fruit		
Vegetable		
Fat		

Meal 2	Time:	How do you feel during?
Protein		
Fruit		
Vegetable		
Fat		

Meal 3	Time:	How do you feel after?
Protein		
Fruit		
Vegetable		
Fat		

Snack	Time:
Protein	
Vegetable	

Day 72

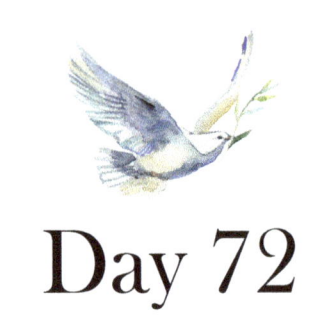

Date: _____

<u>Isaiah 41:10 (NIV)</u>
**So do not fear, for I am with you; do not be dismayed, for I am your God.
I will strengthen you and help you; I will uphold you with my righteous right hand.**

LOOK AT WHAT is promised once you accept Jesus as your savior and begin your journey walking in the purpose God has for you. He is with you every day, every moment, and throughout every decision! No matter what the world will throw at you, God is there. He is ready to guide you, strengthen you, and mold you. I can tell you that only God can deliver the promises in Isaiah.

What do you choose today?
_____
_____
_____

What are you grateful for?
_____
_____
_____

Prayer Request
_____
_____
_____

Food Journal		**Movement**
Water _ _ _ _ _ _ _ _ _ _ _		**HIIT**
Meal 1	Time:	Exercise 1:
Protein		Exercise 2:
Fruit		Exercise 3:
Vegetable		Exercise 4:
Fat		Exercise 5:

Meal 2	Time:	How do you feel before?
Protein		
Fruit		
Vegetable		
Fat		

Meal 3	Time:	How do you feel during?
Protein		
Fruit		
Vegetable		
Fat		

Snack	Time:	How do you feel after?
Protein		
Vegetable		

Day 73

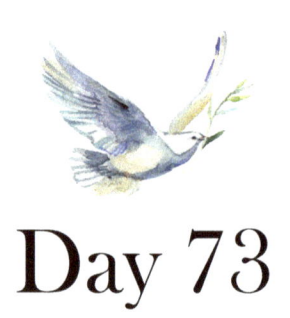

Date: _____

Matthew 11:28 (NIV)

Come to me, all you who are weary and burdened, and I will give you rest. Take my yoke and learn from me, for I am gentle and humble in heart, and you will find rest for your souls.

OUR JOURNEY AS a Christian is not always easy, especially at first. People around you will see a difference. Your friends may make fun of you for not going out to places you once did. Your peers at work may make you the poke of gossip because you no longer engage. It can at times be difficult living the Christian life. Don't be discouraged. Here God tells you he is there to lighten your load. Have faith knowing this new way of walking becomes more joyful because you begin to learn to rest in God. Allow Him to lead you, and you will find His path brings you peace.

Notes from your meditation:

_____
_____
_____

What are you grateful for?

_____
_____
_____

Prayer Request

_____
_____
_____

Food Journal		Movement
Water _ _ _ _ _ _ _ _ _ _ _		**Upper Body:** 3 sets of 12 each exercise
Meal 1	Time:	Exercise 1:
Protein		Exercise 2:
Fruit		Exercise 3:
Vegetable		Exercise 4:
		Exercise 5:
Fat		

Meal 2	Time:	How do you feel before?
Protein		
Fruit		
Vegetable		
Fat		

Meal 3	Time:	How do you feel during?
Protein		
Fruit		
Vegetable		
Fat		

Snack	Time:	How do you feel after?
Protein		
Vegetable		

Day 74

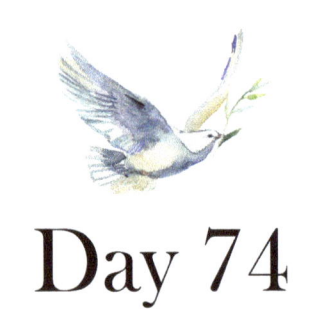

Date: _____

Romans 12:1-2 (NIV)

Therefore, I urge you, brothers and sisters, in view of God's mercy, to offer your bodies as a living sacrifice, holy and pleasing to God—this is your true and proper worship. Do not conform to the pattern of this world but be transformed by the renewing of your mind. Then you will be able to test and approve what God's will is - his good, pleasing, and perfect will.

GOD WANTS US to renew our minds daily. What does this mean? It means begin your day reading the word. Meditate on it and apply it to your daily walk. As the world begins to throw things at you, the power of the Word will rise in you. God's Word gives you tools to help you in your new journey. Do not become what the world wants you to be. This only brings destruction to your mind and body. Shield yourself with the Word of God.

Notes from your meditation:

_____
_____
_____

What are you grateful for?

_____
_____
_____

Prayer Request

_____
_____
_____

Food Journal	**Movement**
Water __ __ __ __ __ __ __ __ __ __	**Cardio** 30 minutes
	What Type:

Meal 1	Time:	How do you feel before?
Protein		
Fruit		
Vegetable		
Fat		

Meal 2	Time:	How do you feel during?
Protein		
Fruit		
Vegetable		
Fat		

Meal 3	Time:	How do you feel after?
Protein		
Fruit		
Vegetable		
Fat		

Snack	Time:
Protein	
Vegetable	

Day 75

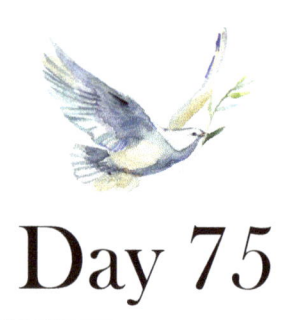

Date: _____

Romans 8:1-2 (NIV)

Therefore, there is now no condemnation for those who are in Christ Jesus, because through Christ Jesus the law of the Spirit who gives life has set you free from the law of sin and death.

THE WORLD ALWAYS wants to condemn and bring us down. So many television programs and social media posts show people's failures. People are always disagreeing with one another and chastising each other. It is refreshing to know there is only One that we need to please. He does not condemn us if we believe and walk in His redemption. We are free from the world. It takes time walking with God daily to fully grasp this concept. Once understood, the freedom that falls over you is amazing.

Yes, you will fall, but does it really matter if you are truly trying to walk in the purpose of God. God knows your heart and is ready to forgive and help you move forward.

How often do you chastise someone undeservedly? Can you help others as they are learning to walk in Christ? Can you show others the mercy God shows you?

_____
_____
_____
_____

What are you grateful for?

_____
_____
_____

Prayer Request

_____
_____
_____

Food Journal		Movement
Water _ _ _ _ _ _ _ _ _ _ _ _		**HIIT**
Meal 1	Time:	Exercise 1:
Protein		Exercise 2:
		Exercise 3:
Fruit		Exercise 4:
Vegetable		Exercise 5:
Fat		

Meal 2	Time:	How do you feel before?
Protein		
Fruit		
Vegetable		
Fat		

Meal 3	Time:	How do you feel during?
Protein		
Fruit		
Vegetable		
Fat		

Snack	Time:	How do you feel after?
Protein		
Vegetable		

Day 76

Date: _____

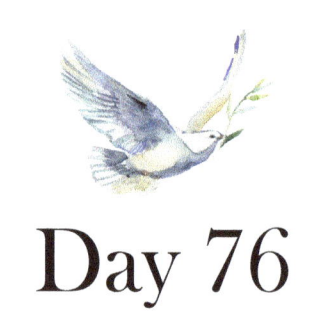

Romans 8:5-8 (NIV)

Those who live according to the flesh have their minds set on what the flesh desires; but those who live in accordance with the Spirit have their minds set on what the Spirit desires. The mind governed by the Spirit is life and peace. The mind governed by the flesh is hostile to God; it does not submit to God's law, nor can it do so. Those who are in the realm of the flesh cannot please God.

THIS VERSE WILL begin to move you. How often do we as humans want to have worldly things. We desire beautiful homes, lavish vacations, jewelry, clothing, spa treatments, and a list that goes on and on. I am not saying these things are evil. I am saying if we put these things as priorities and live by these fleshly desires, we are not doing what God wants us to do. If we spend money we do not have, we are not being good stewards of our finances. If we neglect what God wants us to be doing and instead do what we desire constantly, we are not living within the Spirit's desires. First seek God.

Are you in debt? Do you choose lavish vacations when you can only afford to go close to home and for a less amount of time? Do you have a closet full of clothes that you do not wear. When you are not helping the church, feeding the poor, teaching the scripture, and using the talents God gave you, then you are not living by the Spirit's desires. When we chase dreams that do not line up with God's word, we are not living the desires of the Spirit. He knows your heart and wants to bless you, but we must be able to make wise decisions. HE will only give us what we are capable of managing wisely.

Take a self-inventory here. Do not be ashamed God is not condemning you, He is enlightening you.

_____
_____
_____

What are you grateful for?

_____
_____
_____

Prayer Request

_____
_____
_____

Food Journal		**Movement**
Water _ _ _ _ _ _ _ _ _ _		**Lower Body:** 3 sets of 12 each exercise
Meal 1	Time:	Exercise 1:
Protein		Exercise 2:
Fruit		Exercise 3:
Vegetable		Exercise 4:
Fat		Exercise 5:

Meal 2	Time:	How do you feel before?
Protein		
Fruit		
Vegetable		
Fat		

Meal 3	Time:	How do you feel during?
Protein		
Fruit		
Vegetable		
Fat		

Snack	Time:	How do you feel after?
Protein		
Vegetable		

Day 77

Date: _____

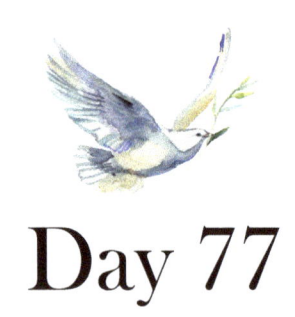

Romans 8:18 (NIV)
I consider that our present sufferings are not worth comparing with the glory that will be revealed in us.

THERE WILL BE times when we feel we are suffering. We may even suffer at times for Christ. The disciples surely did. However, life in eternity with God is far better than what this earth can provide. Do not compare today to your eternity. Live today walking with Christ. Rest in Him knowing that He is creating in you a warrior, a teacher, a host to provide shelter, or possibly a refuge for the weak. Be open to what God will do in you. Be ready to live like you never expected you would.

How do you desire to live? Does this desire line up with the word?

_____
_____
_____

What are you grateful for?

_____
_____
_____

Prayer Request

_____
_____
_____

Food Journal	Movement
Water __ __ __ __ __ __ __ __ __ __ __ __	**Rest Day**
	You can do Active Rest

Meal 1	Time:	
Protein		Walk at a slow pace.
Fruit		Low impact hiking
Vegetable		Low impact biking
Fat		

Meal 2	Time:	How do you feel before?
Protein		
Fruit		
Vegetable		
Fat		

Meal 3	Time:	How do you feel during?
Protein		
Fruit		
Vegetable		
Fat		

Snack	Time:	How do you feel after?
Protein		
Vegetable		

Day 78

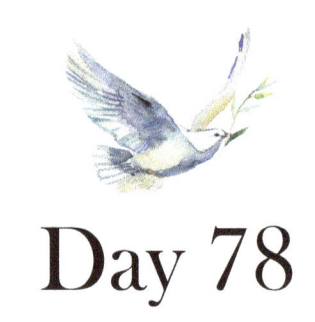

Date: _____

Romans 8:28 (NIV)
And we know that in all things God works for the good of those who love him, who have been called according to his purpose.

GOD CREATED EACH person with a purpose. It is up to us as individuals to follow Him. He knows we are sinners and that we will fall. If we submit to Him, He will make our disasters turn into something for His glory. There are countless couples that have survived adultery. There are many who have been addicts that God has helped through recovery. There are people that have lied, gossiped, stolen things, and even physically hurt others that God has helped. He can turn anyone that dedicates their life to God into a disciple for Him. He can use your past to show that it does not matter where you are in life, God meets you there, dusts you off, and helps you overcome what the enemy has tried to destroy. Do not be overcome with guilt and shame for things you did before you began your journey. You are forgiven if you just ask.

What do you feel you have not let go of? What do you feel you need help with?

_____
_____
_____

What are you grateful for?

_____
_____
_____

Prayer Request

_____
_____
_____

Food Journal	**Movement**
Water __ __ __ __ __ __ __ __ __ __	**Cardio** 30 minutes
	What Type:

Meal 1	Time:	How do you feel before?
Protein		
Fruit		
Vegetable		
Fat		

Meal 2	Time:	How do you feel during?
Protein		
Fruit		
Vegetable		
Fat		

Meal 3	Time:	How do you feel after?
Protein		
Fruit		
Vegetable		
Fat		

Snack	Time:	
Protein		
Vegetable		

Day 79

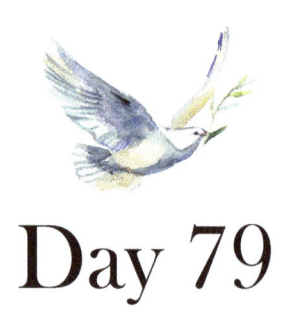

Date: _____

1 John 4:16-17 (NIV)

And so we know and rely on the love God has for us. God is love. Whoever lives in love lives in God, and God in them. This is how love is made complete among us so that we will have confidence on the Day of judgement: in this world we are like Jesus.

GOD IS LOVE. Each day we walk in his love, we should try to be more like Jesus. We need to be working on laying ourselves down and picking Him up. This begins with love. There are people in your life that will test this love daily. That is life. It is our job to be in prayer for those people. Ask God to love them through you. This can be a challenge some days. However, the good thing about God's love is He will forgive. Make sure you take challenges to God as they arise. Be willing to ask Him and the person you may not have shown love to for forgiveness. This is a very powerful healing. Don't worry. You will get stronger each day if you are willing to walk in your purpose.

Where can you show more love in your daily walk?

_____
_____
_____

What are you grateful for?

_____
_____
_____

Prayer Request

_____
_____
_____

Food Journal		**Movement**
Water _ _ _ _ _ _ _ _ _ _ _ _		**HIIT**
Meal 1	Time:	Exercise 1:
Protein		Exercise 2:
		Exercise 3:
Fruit		Exercise 4:
Vegetable		Exercise 5:
Fat		

Meal 2	Time:	How do you feel before?
Protein		
Fruit		
Vegetable		
Fat		

Meal 3	Time:	How do you feel during?
Protein		
Fruit		
Vegetable		
Fat		

Snack	Time:	How do you feel after?
Protein		
Vegetable		

Day 80

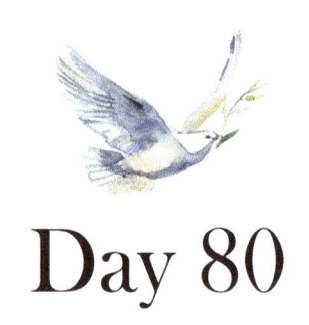

Date: _____

Ephesians 4:22-24 (NIV)

You were taught, with regard to your former way of life, to put off your old self, which is being corrupted by its deceitful desires; to be made new in the attitude of your minds; and to put on the new self, created to be like God in true righteousness and holiness.

BEFORE YOU SUBMITTED your life to God you had a different way of thinking. Your thought process was selfish and self-centered. You were in the world and focused on what it had to offer. Today, 80 days of beginning your day in the Word I am certain your thought process has changed a bit. I hope you have begun to put others before yourself. You are stopping and thinking through tasks before you begin them. I pray if you have been living in anxiety and strife these emotions have changed to joy and peace. God knows your journey will not be perfect. His desire is that each day you strive to be better than the day before. Always work towards being more in His image.

Notes on your meditation:
_____
_____
_____

What are you grateful for?
_____
_____
_____

Prayer Request
_____
_____
_____

Food Journal		**Movement**
Water __ __ __ __ __ __ __ __ __ __		**Upper Body:** 3 sets of 12 each exercise
Meal 1	Time:	Exercise 1:
Protein		Exercise 2:
		Exercise 3:
Fruit		Exercise 4:
Vegetable		Exercise 5:
Fat		

Meal 2	Time:	How do you feel before?
Protein		
Fruit		
Vegetable		
Fat		

Meal 3	Time:	How do you feel during?
Protein		
Fruit		
Vegetable		
Fat		

Snack	Time:	How do you feel after?
Protein		
Vegetable		

Day 81

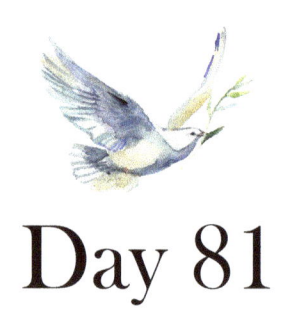

Date: _____

Daniel 12:3 (NIV)
Those who are wise will shine like the brightness of the heavens, and those who lead many to righteousness, like the stars forever and ever.

WE ARE SO precious to God. The Bible is not a rule book written with the intention of removing fun from our lives. It is a guide that was written to prevent the world's sin and influence from creating destruction in our lives. Being wise and having this wonderful tool helps you shine in this world. The joy that flows through you will make others want what you have which will lead others to God.

Be wise today and walk tall in the Lord.
Have you seen a change in your daily attitude over the past few months? Do you feel a new joy rising in you?

_____
_____
_____

What are you grateful for?

_____
_____
_____

Prayer Request

_____
_____
_____

Food Journal		**Movement**
Water _ _ _ _ _ _ _ _ _ _ _ _		**Cardio** 30 minutes
		What Type:

Meal 1	Time:	How do you feel before?
Protein		
Fruit		
Vegetable		
Fat		

Meal 2	Time:	How do you feel during?
Protein		
Fruit		
Vegetable		
Fat		

Meal 3	Time:	How do you feel after?
Protein		
Fruit		
Vegetable		
Fat		

Snack	Time:
Protein	
Vegetable	

A DAILY WALK IN THE TEMPLE

Day 82

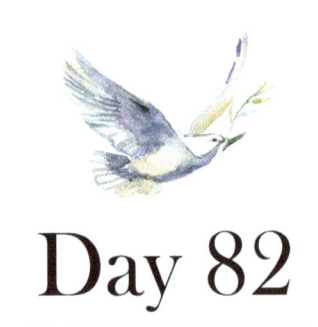

Date: _____

Romans 12:21 (NIV)
Do not be overcome by evil but overcome evil with good.

WHEN YOU WALK daily with God, the Holy Spirit, and Christ your mind begins to change. Your thought process begins to become positive. You start to see the good in people. Life choices start to bring freedom and not destruction. You are becoming life minded and not death minded. You begin to recognize the evil in the world and choose good instead. Your thoughts are shifting from what others are thinking about me to how I can please my Lord and Savior. You allow the Spirit of God to rise in you in difficult times, and when you fall you do not dwell on your failure. You make amends and when necessary, ask God to forgive you. You get up, dust yourself off, and start again.

What have you overcome by making the changes you have made over the past few months?

_____
_____
_____

What are you grateful for?

_____
_____
_____

Prayer Request

_____
_____
_____

Food Journal		Movement	
Water _ _ _ _ _ _ _ _ _ _ _		**HIIT**	
Meal 1	Time:	Exercise 1:	
Protein		Exercise 2:	
		Exercise 3:	
Fruit		Exercise 4:	
Vegetable		Exercise 5:	
Fat			

Meal 2	Time:	How do you feel before?
Protein		
Fruit		
Vegetable		
Fat		

Meal 3	Time:	How do you feel during?
Protein		
Fruit		
Vegetable		
Fat		

Snack	Time:	How do you feel after?
Protein		
Vegetable		

Day 83

Date: _____

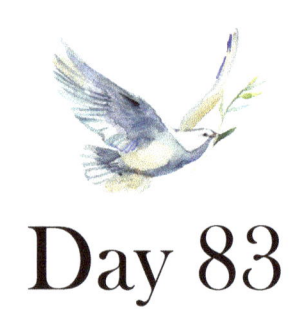

1 John 5:4-5 (NIV)

For everyone born of God overcomes the world. This is the victory that has overcome the world, even our faith. Who is it that overcomes the world? Only the one who believes that Jesus is the Son of God.

IF YOU ARE here on day 83, I want to believe you have accepted Christ as your Savior. If not, I invite you to become a brother or sister in Christ with me. You are an overcomer. With the Spirit of God dwelling in your temple you will overcome eternal death. Each day make the decision to rise in Christ. Immerse yourself in the Word and follow God's purpose you are hiding in your heart. Fill yourself with truth and goodness. Be an overcomer with me today. You will have days that will be more difficult than others. Knowing that you have a power in you that can lift you and guide you through those days is much better than being alone. Praise God!

Notes on your meditation:
_____
_____
_____

What are you grateful for?
_____
_____
_____

Prayer Request
_____
_____
_____

Food Journal		**Movement**
Water _ _ _ _ _ _ _ _ _ _ _ _ _ _		**Lower Body:** 3 sets of 12 each exercise
Meal 1	Time:	Exercise 1: Exercise 2: Exercise 3: Exercise 4: Exercise 5:
Protein		
Fruit		
Vegetable		
Fat		

Meal 2	Time:	How do you feel before?
Protein		
Fruit		
Vegetable		
Fat		

Meal 3	Time:	How do you feel during?
Protein		
Fruit		
Vegetable		
Fat		

Snack	Time:	How do you feel after?
Protein		
Vegetable		

Day 84

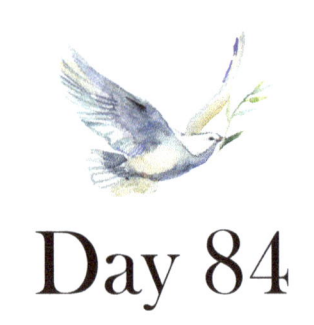

Date: _____

Psalms 3:3 (NIV)
But you, LORD, are a shield around me, my glory, the One who lifts my head high.

YESTERDAY, WE READ we are overcomers if we accept Christ as our Savior. Today we see God is our shield and glory. We have an invisible barrier of shields around us to protect us. We stand in His glory. We can call on God to help us out of dangers or prevent us from walking into dangers. We walk according to God's and He helps us make better decisions. Each morning ask God to help you see where you should walk, to give you the words when you should speak, and to help you be still when you should just listen.

I can recall countless times when I decided to do things that were worldly and found trouble. Now, I try my best to think, look, and listen before I step or speak. I want to glorify God and walk with the One who lifts my head high.

How often do you move or speak and find destruction?

What are you grateful for?

_____
_____
_____

Prayer Request

_____
_____
_____

Food Journal	**Movement**
Water _ _ _ _ _ _ _ _ _ _	**Rest Day**
	You can do Active Rest

Meal 1	Time:	
Protein		Walk at a slow pace.
Fruit		Low impact hiking
Vegetable		Low impact biking
Fat		

Meal 2	Time:	How do you feel before?
Protein		
Fruit		
Vegetable		
Fat		

Meal 3	Time:	How do you feel during?
Protein		
Fruit		
Vegetable		
Fat		

Snack	Time:	How do you feel after?
Protein		
Vegetable		

Day 85

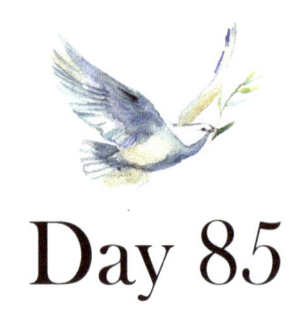

Date: _____

1 John 1:5 (NIV)
This is the message we have heard from him and declare to you: God is light; in him there is no darkness at all.

THE LIGHT IS God's Spirit in you. You take this light out into the world every day. Shining joy and peace to anyone that is near you. You bring the light to the world carrying Jesus everywhere you go. You will not be overcome by the world. Jesus has already won the war. Just walk in peace daily with Him. Know that we will have the ultimate eternal life. One day we will live where there is no darkness at all.

How can you be the light today for someone walking in darkness?

_____
_____
_____

What are you grateful for?

_____
_____
_____

Prayer Request

_____
_____
_____

Food Journal	Movement
Water _ _ _ _ _ _ _ _ _ _ _ _	**Cardio** 30 minutes
	What Type:

Meal 1	Time:	How do you feel before?
Protein		
Fruit		
Vegetable		
Fat		

Meal 2	Time:	How do you feel during?
Protein		
Fruit		
Vegetable		
Fat		

Meal 3	Time:	How do you feel after?
Protein		
Fruit		
Vegetable		
Fat		

Snack	Time:
Protein	
Vegetable	

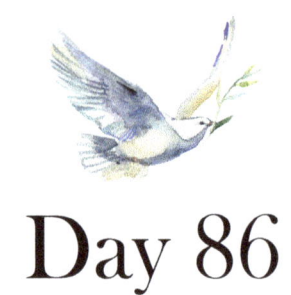

Day 86

Date: _____

John 13:35 (NIV)
By this everyone will know that you are my disciples if you love one another."

Love
Do you really know what love is?

Self-love:
Do you love yourself the way you were created? He didn't make a mistake. If we cannot love ourselves, how can we love others?

Love your enemy:
Well, this is not easy. We are to love those that oppose us and allow God to deal with them. HE can help them change or take care of the situation. It is our job to love them and let Him.

Love your family: Sometimes our family is the most difficult to love. We do not choose our family. They are the ones that usually stay in our lives. They know our weaknesses better than our enemies and at times push those boundaries further than anyone else will. Yet, we are to love them regardless.

PLEASE UNDERSTAND THAT loving others does not mean you should be a door mat. Sometimes we need to love from afar until God releases you to return. Love may mean to get out of God's way while He does His job.

Love others today and allow God to discipline or give mercy as needed. Let God rebuild or take away. Your job is to LOVE.

What are you grateful for?

_____
_____
_____

Prayer Request

_____
_____
_____

Food Journal		Movement
Water _ _ _ _ _ _ _ _ _ _ _		**HIIT**
Meal 1	Time:	Exercise 1:
Protein		Exercise 2:
		Exercise 3:
Fruit		Exercise 4:
Vegetable		Exercise 5:
Fat		

Meal 2	Time:	How do you feel before?
Protein		
Fruit		
Vegetable		
Fat		

Meal 3	Time:	How do you feel during?
Protein		
Fruit		
Vegetable		
Fat		

Snack	Time:	How do you feel after?
Protein		
Vegetable		

Day 87

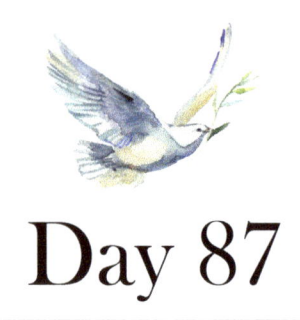

Date: _____

Psalms 139:14 (NIV)
**I praise you because I am fearfully and wonderfully made;
your works are wonderful I know that full well.**

AS WE COME to the end of your first 90 days of walking in the temple you should know that you were fearfully and wonderfully created by the Master. The Father created you in love. You were made perfect in His eyes. Do not be ashamed of who you are. Make each day better than the day before. Become the person you were created to be. Lay the things of the world down so you can pick up the talents God gave you to use for His kingdom.

Today amp up what you have been doing to this point. Stay in prayer longer, give more mercy to those around you, eat a little cleaner, and move with more intensity.

Notes on your meditation:
_____
_____
_____

What are you grateful for?
_____
_____
_____

Prayer Request
_____
_____
_____

Food Journal		**Movement**
Water _ _ _ _ _ _ _ _ _ _		**Upper Body:** 3 sets of 12 each exercise
Meal 1	Time:	Exercise 1:
Protein		Exercise 2:
Fruit		Exercise 3:
Vegetable		Exercise 4:
		Exercise 5:
Fat		

Meal 2	Time:	How do you feel before?
Protein		
Fruit		
Vegetable		
Fat		

Meal 3	Time:	How do you feel during?
Protein		
Fruit		
Vegetable		
Fat		

Snack	Time:	How do you feel after?
Protein		
Vegetable		

Day 88

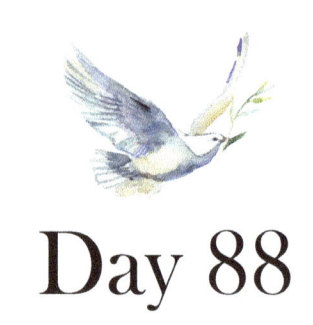

Date: _____

Ephesians 2:10 (NIV)
For we are God's handiwork, created in Christ Jesus to do good works, which God prepared in advance for us to do.

TODAY TAKE TIME to analyze your life to this point. Look at how beautifully you were created. What talents you were given? What are your strengths? What do you feel you are led to do for Him?

Write all this down and create a plan to fulfill what you are led to do. Once you have a plan, pray over it. Ask God to lead you and give you wisdom, knowledge, and strength to walk it out. Ask God to go before you and make a path to walk tall and fulfill what you were created to do.

What are your strengths and talents?
_____
_____
_____

What do you feel God is leading you to do?
_____
_____
_____

Begin your plan:
_____
_____
_____
_____
_____
_____
_____

Food Journal	Movement
Water __ __ __ __ __ __ __ __ __ __	**Cardio** 30 minutes
	What Type:

Meal 1	Time:	How do you feel before?
Protein		
Fruit		
Vegetable		
Fat		

Meal 2	Time:	How do you feel during?
Protein		
Fruit		
Vegetable		
Fat		

Meal 3	Time:	How do you feel after?
Protein		
Fruit		
Vegetable		
Fat		

Snack	Time:
Protein	
Vegetable	

Day 89

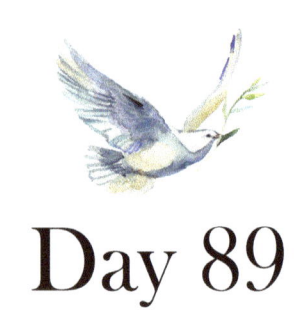

Date: _____

1 Samuel 16:7 (NIV)

But the LORD said to *Samuel*, "Do not consider his appearance or his height, for I have rejected him. The LORD does not look at the things people look at. People look at the outward appearance, but the LORD looks at the heart."

EATING CLEAN AND working out is not for our outward appearance. When we do these things, we are healing our bodies. Yes, we do feel emotionally better when our outward appearance looks nice; however, creating a temple to be able to serve the Lord is the ultimate reason we eat clean and move. God does not want us to be obsessed with how we look or what we wear. He wants us to be healthy from the inside out, beginning with our spiritual life. If we are working towards cleaning our life up, we should be seeing our mind and body following this path as well.

Look at your heart. How are you living and loving?

Notes on your meditation:

_____
_____
_____

What are you grateful for?

_____
_____
_____

Prayer Request

_____
_____
_____

Food Journal			Movement
Water _ _ _ _ _ _ _ _ _ _ _ _			**HIIT**
Meal 1	Time:		Exercise 1:
Protein			Exercise 2:
			Exercise 3:
Fruit			Exercise 4:
Vegetable			Exercise 5:
Fat			

Meal 2	Time:	How do you feel before?
Protein		
Fruit		
Vegetable		
Fat		

Meal 3	Time:	How do you feel during?
Protein		
Fruit		
Vegetable		
Fat		

Snack	Time:	How do you feel after?
Protein		
Vegetable		

Day 90

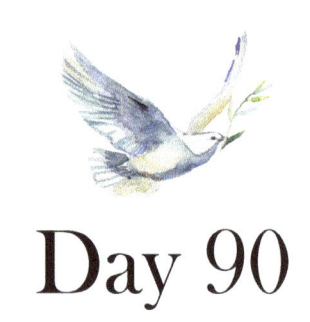

Date: _____

Genesis 1:27 (NIV)
So, God created mankind in his own image, in the image of God he created them; male and female he created them.

WE ARE CREATED to be like the perfect One. We are created to be whole. We should be walking in the Spirit. We have to live our lives to be able to walk out our purpose. The only way we can walk out our purpose is to read the word, stay in prayer, and take care of our bodies. This is how we will endure until the end.

Over the past 90 days where have you changed the most?
_____
_____
_____

What are you grateful for?
_____
_____
_____

What prayer requests have been answered?
_____
_____
_____

Did you create a plan to walk with God daily?
_____
_____
_____

Food Journal	**Movement**
Water _ _ _ _ _ _ _ _ _ _ _ _	**Lower Body:** 3 sets of 12 each exercise

Meal 1	Time:	Exercise 1:
Protein		Exercise 2:
Fruit		Exercise 3:
Vegetable		Exercise 4:
Fat		Exercise 5:

Meal 2	Time:	How do you feel before?
Protein		
Fruit		
Vegetable		
Fat		

Meal 3	Time:	How do you feel during?
Protein		
Fruit		
Vegetable		
Fat		

Snack	Time:	How do you feel after?
Protein		
Vegetable		

Thank you

God, I want to thank you first for pushing me to get out of my box. I feel like Moses did when you called him to speak. You have led me through my entire life to this point.

I want to say a special thank you to a few people who have been on this journey with me. First and foremost, I want to thank my parents. Parenting is difficult at best, but with a strong-willed child like me I am sure you both had a few struggles.

A special thanks to my brother Bobby. I have always admired and looked up to you.

I would like to thank my husband. You have been by my side for the past 32 years and have never left me. You have helped me find my way through the dark and now we are walking in God's will. For this I am truly grateful.

I also want to thank my daughter. You have always been a true gift. You have supported me in my wellness journey from Day one when I decided to go back to school and get my certifications.

Thank you to all my friends. I cannot tell you how much your responses to my devotions have meant to me. When you tell me something spoke to you, I knew God was at work.

Lastly, I want to thank each of you that purchased this journal.

Thank you for your commitment to live a life with God.